A HUMANE VISION OF CLINICAL PSYCHOLOGY, VOLUME I

The primary purpose of psychotherapy is to improve a patient's subjective experience. *A Humane Vision of Clinical Psychology, Volume I* shows readers what this might really mean and where prevailing views go wrong in achieving it.

In so doing, the text lays out an alternative idea of human suffering and human healing, one that deemphasizes constructs and prioritizes experience itself. Early chapters argue that helping people to "know new things" is the ultimate target of psychotherapeutic change, but that contemporary clinical psychology has not sufficiently reflected on the complications of this task. A theory is then offered, which suggests that the unthinkable aspects of human experience are responsible for the very ways in which we human beings think. From there, the book invites and outlines a serious reformulation of psychotherapy in which human cognition is not the seat but the beneficiary of human change.

A Humane Vision will be valuable for therapists, psychologists, psychiatrists, and other practitioners as well as graduate and undergraduate students in the fields of psychiatry, psychology, psychotherapy, mental health, social work, and philosophy. It will be of great interest for clinicians who find themselves disenchanted with the field's current ethos, which is stilted by scientistic approaches to soothing the suffering of the other.

Robert A. Graceffo, PhD, is a clinical psychologist in private practice and a lecturer and supervisor in the psychiatry department at Harvard Medical School, USA.

ADVANCES IN THEORETICAL AND PHILOSOPHICAL PSYCHOLOGY

Series Editor
Brent D. Slife
Brigham Young University

From Scientific Psychology to the Study of Persons: A Psychologist's Memoir
Jack Martin

Problematic Research Practices and Inertia in Scientific Psychology: History, Sources, and Recommended Solutions
James T. Lamiell and Kathleen L. Slaney

Critical Psychology Praxis: Psychosocial Non-Alignment to Modernity/Coloniality
Robert K. Beshara

Global Pandemics and Epistemic Crises in Psychology: A Socio-Philosophical Approach
Martin Dege and Irene Strasser

Hermeneutic Dialogue and Shaping the Landscape of Theoretical and Philosophical Psychology: The Work of Frank Richardson
Robert C. Bishop

A Humane Vision of Clinical Psychology, Volume 1
The Theoretical Basis for a Compassionate Psychotherapy
Robert A. Graceffo

A Humane Vision of Clinical Psychology, Volume 2
Explorations into the Practice of Compassionate Psychotherapy
Robert A. Graceffo

https://www.routledge.com/psychology/series/TPP

A HUMANE VISION OF CLINICAL PSYCHOLOGY, VOLUME I

The Theoretical Basis for a Compassionate Psychotherapy

Robert A. Graceffo

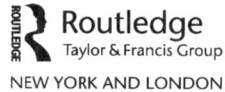

Routledge
Taylor & Francis Group

NEW YORK AND LONDON

Cover image: © Getty Images

First published 2022
by Routledge
605 Third Avenue, New York, NY 10158

and by Routledge
4 Park Square, Milton Park, Abingdon, Oxon OX14 4RN

Routledge is an imprint of the Taylor & Francis Group, an informa business

Library of Congress Cataloging-in-Publication Data
A catalog record for this title has been requested

ISBN: 978-1-032-30481-6 (hbk)
ISBN: 978-1-032-25992-5 (pbk)
ISBN: 978-1-003-30528-6 (ebk)

DOI: 10.4324/9781003305286

Typeset in Bembo
by Taylor & Francis Books

For East Genesee Street, where great aunts were more like saints, cousins were more like brothers and sisters, brothers were more like eager accomplices, and sisters were more like wise, older teachers; where parents served as exemplars of The Good; and where, despite all my education and fancy degrees and titles, I learned everything I ever really needed.

For the intuitive ones, who have always understood more than they've had any reason to, and often more than they could say; and who protect the spirit of this field during a time in which it needs protecting.

Most of all, for my wife, Samantha, whose gift for loving defies my words and soothes my soul.

Note: the details of the case illustrations throughout Volume I and Volume II have been altered in ways that ensure confidentiality and make patient identities entirely unknowable.

CONTENTS

ILLUSTRATIONS

Figure

Tables

ACKNOWLEDGMENTS

I need to thank everyone in and around this field who has helped me, professionally, personally, or both. This group includes University of Toledo's Psychological Assessment Lab and everyone in it; the entire Psychology Department at SUNY Brockport; clinical supervisors with whom I thought and talked and debated and wondered, while training in the Harvard Medical School's pre- and post-doc psychology programs (Jack Beinashowitz, Rudy Blier, Chris Bullock, Adam Conklin, Elizabeth Corpt, Rebecca Drill, Jim Feldman, Ramon Greenberg, Linda Luz-Alterman, Al Margulies, Irene Merwin, Chris Morse, Humphrey Morris, Elizabeth Schatzel-Murphy, Alan Siegel, and June Wolf); beloved colleagues I met at different Boston hospitals who enriched my work in one way or another (Dan and Katy, Heidi Thermenos, Sarah Keenan, Cheskie Rosenzweig, and Shelisa Ramsammy, among others); and my MA and PhD advisors (Jan Gillespie, Greg Meyer, and Joni Mihura). A special thanks to Joni, whose authenticity in both mentorship and friendship served only to strengthen my most natural clinical impulse: that in order to be useful to the other, we must be ourselves with them.

I would also like to thank Jamie, an archetypal partner-in-crime for the ages. The same good nature, wit, and absurdist humor that once made him just the right companion for an odyssey into the strange world of clinical psychology now make him a clinician of special talents, and a breath of fresh air to his patients in numbers untold.

In addition, thank you to Matthew Johnson, who did me the favor of carefully reading a long manuscript and providing very thoughtful feedback.

Finally, I would like to thank Brent Slife, the editor of this book series, for his interest in my work, and all the Routledge staff with whom I had the pleasure of working on this project. I am very grateful that these books found the right home.

ADVANCES IN THEORETICAL AND PHILOSOPHICAL PSYCHOLOGY: SERIES FOREWORD

Brent D. Slife, Editor

Psychologists need to face the facts. Their commitment to empiricism for answering disciplinary questions does not prevent pivotal questions from arising that cannot be evaluated exclusively through empirical methods, hence the title of this series: *Advances in Theoretical and Philosophical Psychology*. For example, such moral questions as, "What is the nature of a good life?" are crucial to psychotherapists but are not answerable through empirical methods alone. And what of the methods themselves? Many have worried that our current psychological means of investigation are not adequate for fully understanding the person (e.g., Gantt & Williams, 2018; Schiff, 2019). How do we address this concern through empirical methods without running headlong into the dilemma of methods investigating themselves? Such questions are in some sense philosophical, to be sure, but the discipline of psychology cannot advance even its own empirical agenda without addressing questions like these in defensible ways.

How then should the discipline of psychology deal with such distinctly theoretical questions? We could leave the answers exclusively to professional philosophers, but this option would mean that the conceptual foundations of the discipline, including the conceptual framework of empiricism itself, are left to scholars who are *outside* the discipline. As undoubtedly helpful as philosophers are and will be, this situation would mean that the people doing the actual psychological work, psychologists themselves, are divorced from the people who formulate and re-formulate the conceptual foundations of that work. This division of labor would not seem to serve the long-term viability of the discipline.

Instead, the founders of psychology—thinkers such as Wundt, Freud, and James—recognized the importance of psychologists in formulating their own foundations. These parents of psychology not only did their own theorizing, in cooperation with many other disciplines; they also realized the significance of psychologists continuously *re*-examining these theories and philosophies. This re-examination process allowed for the people most directly involved in and knowledgeable about the discipline to be the ones to decide *what* changes were needed, and *how* such changes would best be implemented. This book series is dedicated to that task: the examining and re-examining of psychology's foundations.

References

Gantt, E., & Williams, R. (2018). *On hijacking science: Exploring the nature and consequences of overreach in psychology*. London: Routledge.
Schiff, B. (2019). *Situating qualitative methods in psychological science*. London: Routledge.

PREFACE

I have written and rewritten this book in my mind, dozens and dozens of times. For years, the bulk of my mental energy was aimed at the same set of ideas. I turned them over relentlessly, apprehending them from different angles and touching their assorted contours. Over time, these ideas began to take the shape of something like a philosophy about people and the world. This vision of human life, when I finally gripped it completely, impacted my own in every possible way. I found myself not just conceiving of the world differently but being differently in the world. I was moved to new pursuits, entirely. Eventually, I spent a decade ensuring that my life and work followed from that which I came to so sincerely believe.

In a certain sense, my personal development and the central themes that grow through this text bear no important distinction, which poses some difficulty in characterizing the book. It is at once a personal reflection, a theory, and an argument. Maybe it's more an argument than anything. However, while I want to convince you, my only real claim about everything that follows is this: it is what I have come to know. It isn't absolute truth, it isn't morally better, and it isn't a 1:1 depiction of reality (despite the periodic insistence with which I will certainly present my views). This book represents only what I have seen as I have looked around this world—nothing more. In this way, it is more a vision than a proof. It is important for me to say so at the outset because I spend a lot of time claiming that knowledge is what the knower makes of the world. This claim so too applies to me, absolutely and without exception, as I make assertions throughout this book.

Regardless of how the book is best characterized, however, its subject matter is less up for debate. This is a book about love. The meaning of love, as I am interested in it, is a bit different than how it tends to be colloquially rendered, in that it is single-minded and purposeful. Loving, as I mean it, aspires exclusively to heal. And this raises the first of many questions I will ask the reader to think about: what is healing? To answer it, we must first ask another one: what is harm? Now we have two questions, and we need to see that our answer to the first hinges on our answer to the second. Any process of healing is defined by a kind of restorative effect; therefore, any notion of healing that has ever been offered is linked with an associated and underlying notion of injury, whether explicitly or implicitly, and whether the person doing the offering knows it or not. That is, restoring *what?* This necessary, two-sides-of-the-same-coin relationship that healing has with harm is uniquely relevant to psychotherapy—and particularly, to the psychotherapist.

These days, the obedient clinician knows such things by looking to that which the established order has bestowed from on high—from the perch of empiricism. Let me illustrate this by way of a hypothetical conversation between a *thinking person in 2022* and *the year 2022.*

A THINKING PERSON IN 2022: "What is human harm, injury, and suffering? And what is healing? These are very complicated questions, aren't they? Or, at least, they could be if one really thought hard about it, right?"

2022: "That's easy! Ever hear of Science?"(now noticing a burgeoning sense of pride, but terror too, after having so freely uttered the name of their God).

A THINKING PERSON IN 2022: "Yes, 2022, I've heard of science."

2022: "Okay then, what do the data say? That's where you'll find the answers you seek."

A THINKING PERSON IN 2022: "Okay, but I'm just curious. What do you think? How would one person help another person to develop a healthier psyche?"

2022: "What do you mean, what do I think? There is no need to think anymore. What are you, a dinosaur? Just go find the best protocol and let the intervening begin. Lucky for you, all of human life has already been operationalized and made sense of. Now, get out there and get to work! There are lots of syndromes in need of science-supported behavioral technologies!"

A THINKING PERSON IN 2022: "Do you mean there are lots of people in need of another, caring person?"

2022: "I guess you really are a dinosaur."

I hope my portrayal above is amusing; unfortunately, it can't be *merely amusing* because it is also reflective of reality—a sad one. Many people accept without reservation all that 2022 offers. This is a problem, however, because what could it mean to accept something in the total absence of critical consideration? As science goes, it was never supposed to be a religion, right? Some might say it *cannot* be one. But why not? I am not a person who uses this word in a pejorative way, but when we say that something has become "a religion" as a means of criticizing it, we mean that its followers are unable or unwilling to weigh alternatives. It means thought has stopped. Yet, the situation in which we now find ourselves will turn out to be worse than that; eventually, it will be one in which thought never started.

People born today will never find a world that contains alternatives to the grand operationalization of everything, which means they should not be faulted for accepting this procedure wholesale, as there will be nothing else to consider. Think of it: you've never gone out of your way to find alternatives to breathing oxygen because oxygen is the only game in town. Consequently, you probably don't have much understanding of the most intricate, inner workings of oxygenation. And fair enough. Why would you? You have exactly zero reasons to understand this process precisely for the fact of its real and genuine monopoly. Because there *really aren't* other ways to breathe, an improved comprehension of the only way that exists would be, practically speaking, useless. It would do nothing to incrementally change your life, for better or worse. Understand it or don't; it doesn't matter.

This is precisely where we are in 2022, when it comes to science. Most people don't really know how to think about it, or even that they could, and they certainly don't know how to think about alternatives. As far as most are concerned, science *just is* the method of knowing in the same way oxygen *just is* the molecule for breathing. To be clear—and I will reiterate this throughout the text—my claim is not that the products of science are inherently wrong or useless or anything of the sort. I am certainly not anti-science. I am just strongly pro-thought, pro-critical thought, and even pro-unpopular thought, should it help us move away from reflexive acceptance and toward truth. As a psychologist, my criticism is not with science per se, but with the crippling effect science has had on my field's capacity to think about its work.

At this point, the problem with the hypothetical conversation above should be clear. In contemporary life, a person's belief that science has uncovered the mechanisms of human healing *could be* a product of fair, deliberate, and effortful consideration—and for some, it surely is. But in 2022, this is the exception. It is much more likely that a science devotee is obstructed from the very thought that would allow them to consider more, not only about the world but about themselves. So, let's do something about this. Let's reflect with the explicit aim of finding things that are difficult or inconvenient to consider—and let's consider them. This is the first of many times I will ask the reader to join me in this practice. I should note here that not only will this book require thought on the part of the reader; some of that thought might elicit uneasiness about some of our most taken-for-granted givens. Though it does not reflect the book's fundamental spirit, the reader will notice that the author wonders quite frequently whether the emperor is really clothed, after all.

With just a little reflection on the work that we *actually do* as psychotherapists, something immediately reveals itself to us, which is a thorn in the side of what is arguably 2022's most cherished assumption. Whether it makes its way into our awareness (and for the scientifically devout, it might not); and whether we would admit it to our polite and well-behaved colleagues or to the intelligentsia labeled as such for their commitment to "impartial data," no psychologist who has ever sat across from a patient has done so without *very personal ideas* as to what goes wrong with people—personal ideas, not empirical facts. Healing speech, healing behavior, and a healing presence fail even to be concepts without one's own sense as to the nature of human harm. I am far from a critic of this reality. To the contrary, I am critical of efforts to ignore it, and gleefully critical of attempts to refute it.

How is it refuted? Through claims that impartial data lead to impartial treatments to be delivered impartially, in order to remove some syndrome that has been impartially assessed. Those operating from this viewpoint claim that it is science, not personal predilection, that drives their ideas of psychotherapy and their behavior as psychotherapists. But if we can be honest, an investment in science is still an investment, and I've not heard of investments that can be value-free or impartial. Have you? My point is this: as a psychologist, not only is it impossible to sit down across from someone without a guiding perspective as to what goes wrong in human life, but moreover, if you tried to, you would render yourself perfectly useless to the person with whom you find yourself talking. And for some, empiricism might well constitute this guiding perspective, but we ought not claim it was arrived at "impartially." These perspectives about human harm, if we can just briefly be painfully self-aware, do not derive from empirical facts, nor should they. Instead, they grow out of the values to which we subscribe.

This can be considered a blasphemous stance in the modern world, but it shouldn't be. We all have personal perspectives, whether or not we want to admit such a thing amid our field's current culture of objectivity, data, and facts. Thus, it is incumbent on the data-obsessed clinician to think harder about what he or she *really* thinks of human harm, for without one's own understanding, how could a person perform the most intimate, ambiguous, and personal of all known professional tasks? How could one person foster healing in another? We should ask ourselves what *about us* has landed us on empiricism or humanism or anything else for that matter. If we are honest, the vehicle was not journals nor data but our own experiences, our own struggles, our own hearts. We are just dishonest or perhaps insufficiently reflective (first cousins). How else would we fail to see ourselves in our so-called "theoretical orientations?" It's us, after all, who orients to them.

Even the staunchest empiricist seeking to eradicate the bias of the self from every patient interaction has already failed to do so: it is personal factors that have made impartiality and objectivity so important. This raises another point. We can characterize and even justify our work with patients by pointing to our preferred methods, technologies, or theoretical inclinations (e.g., behaviorism or psycho-analysis; humanism or scientism), but we are still only pointing at ourselves because these conceptual schemes are not independent things in themselves. Rather, they are things by which we ourselves have been compelled. Where does that leave us? In a position where we are forced to admit what is so obviously the case, despite our field's willful blindness. Underneath any intervention, model, or tactic to which a therapist subscribes is, inevitably, a therapist—*that* therapist. There is still a self. As we do our jobs, before we are anything else, before we are a psychologist delivering "behavioral technologies," we are a person. And our job is to talk with other persons.

This is the simplest truth of our job. Were we to admit it, we would also see that the arbitrary interventions by which our field feels "therapy" ought to be constituted is not what helps people; or at the very least, we would see that there is much more going on. Shortly thereafter, we would be in just the right position to question the field's grandest fantasy, which goes something like this: what helps the people who come see us is the "delivery of fact-derived interventions." And if the day we began to see all of this was a day we happened to be feeling particularly bold, we might even begin to acknowledge that we ourselves—one half of the dyad—have a much larger role in helping people than scientistic per-spectives, those that cherish "objective interventions," can ever afford.

My view, if it isn't evident, is that we have an essential responsibility to acknowledge our half of the dyad, and to understand what it's doing and why. We must clarify our personal philosophies, ideas, and approaches, independent of—or in addition to—those that prevail. We must understand how we see human harm. Without doing so, how can we do this work? After all, even the most purely intended setting out in good faith to rescue a wayward ship will surely wreck their own, without an intimate understanding of the storm. We as treaters need to grip human injury before we can grip human healing. As far as I can see, this is often how life goes, too. For many people, there is often a storm before the calm.

The story of my life, before anything else, perhaps even singularly, is a story of a person developing a mind that could be of use—first to myself, which was necessary in the beginning, but ultimately and more importantly, to others. Over the course of this book, I will tell this story in the form of a theory. Yet, this text is no memoir, nor is it a self-help book. It is a way of sharing my view of what life is, a view with worthwhile implications (or at least I think so) for the fields tasked with improving lives in modern life: clinical psychology and related disciplines.

Before delving into it, though, I want to tell the reader very frankly about the origins of this book. And this does involve saying a bit about me. Taken together, what follows between here and the next section (*An Introduction to the Book's Broadest Purposes*) is my attempt to trace the course of experience, or at least its highlights, by which I became the kind of person who would write this kind of book. The truth is that I was always becoming that kind of person, just as *all of us* are *always* becoming. In this sense, I could start at any point in my history. But because I want to spare you a full-blown autobiography, let's go right to the time and place where I found myself in the throes of what I would now call spiritual unease.

Thinking, Thinking, and Thinking

It was seventeen years ago, and I was sitting in a café in New York City. I had just graduated college and spent much of my time exercising in a manner so aggressive as to elicit concern on the faces of fellow gym-goers and runners. Let me say that more plainly: I horrified people. I wish I was exaggerating, but I'm not. On this particular day, I had probably lifted weights in the morning, run somewhere between five and 15 miles in the early afternoon, and then stopped for some food before I would wait tables at 4 pm. I also remember that it was April.

I was eating a sandwich and drinking a coffee when a few guys came in. While looking at the chalkboard menu, they started talking to one of the employees, Vince, a guy I chatted with on occasion. I first made his acquaintance when he, a fellow runner, asked me what race I was training for, after seeing me recklessly running about the neighborhood during a blizzard. Much to his surprise, I was training for nothing. I was just out for a brisk and advised-against-by-the-city-government jog. As these guys talked with Vince, it became clear that they knew each other, but I remember feeling from the start that they didn't have his best interest at heart. They seemed rougher than him, and with a little more to prove than could ever possibly end well for guys, but especially guys their age. Vince seemed not to share these qualities. He was mild-mannered, and not in the way where you expect that he might not be when off the clock. He had a gentleness to him.

A few minutes into their conversation, the group began poking fun at Vince's new shoes, calling them "too girly," incidentally, implying that *their shoes* were appropriately girly (this could have been quite a thread from which Vince could return jabs, but he chose not to or didn't see the irony). It was already hard to watch when it quickly became worse. Vince joined the party, mocking his own shoes with a false delight that distracted from his embarrassment. I remember being as impressed as I was bothered by how quickly he manipulated his disappointment. It nearly didn't register on his face; I wondered if it registered to him at all. I noted this powerful yet invisible maneuver. The trio ordered coffees, then left. On the way out, one of them said something to the effect of, "throw out the lady shoes before we go out tonight, Vivian," or it could have been Valerie (I can't remember exactly, but it was a woman's name that started with a V). Because this comment was both disconnected from prior joking and more public—café-goers were within earshot—it carried an undoubtably hostile edge.

At that point, I was ready to head to work, but since I consistently under-estimated how much I needed to eat in order to counterbalance a truly unne-cessary workout regimen, I ordered more food on the way out. While at the counter, I said very casually, "Too girly compared to what?" Vince looked puz-zled and said, "Oh my shoes?"—as if I could have been referencing any other thing on the planet. "Yeah," I said, "they seem okay to me." He looked slightly less puzzled and replied, "Yeah, they're okay." I responded, "Agreed, take it easy." I then headed to work where I would be a waiter for the next eight hours.

The next morning, I was back in the café to order a coffee on my way to the gym. It was empty, except for Vince, who was working the morning shift. As I started to order the largest coffee on the menu, he cut me off. "I gotta ask you something," he said. "Why did you say that yesterday? About my shoes." He was so earnest. I was all too ready to return the favor. "Because you don't need to do that," I said, much too bluntly. "Do what?" asked Vince. Slowed down by his uncertainty, I responded less assuredly, "I didn't think you needed to align with those guys against yourself." "I know," said Vince. My ears perked up when he said *he knew*. I also experienced a vague feeling like something was seriously wrong. He wasn't lying to me, but it made no sense for him to tell me *he knew*. The day before, he didn't give a single sign that he did. If he knew he ought not mock himself, why did he? This bothered me, and probably made a small con-tribution to my abiding wariness of language, which the reader will come to know well. But I was not bothered by him. I was just bothered, which was a common experience for me around that time. I wondered, did he *really know* he didn't need to devalue himself or did he not? I quickly dropped this line of thought in order to avoid a cognitive rabbit hole, mid-conversation. Vince con-tinued, "but they're just shoes and you have to admit that they were kind of weird."

"Careful, I liked them, remember?" I quipped. Vince laughed. I continued, "And you're wearing them again today, so you don't think they're that weird." We then sat down and talked from about 5 to 5:30 am in a nearly empty café, seriously compromising my pull-up routine in the process, which was slated to begin at 5:15 sharp. At this point I was 23 years old, convinced I knew nothing. Yet I found myself making surprisingly strong claims about what I thought I knew with respect to Vince's behavior on the prior day. The case I made, half-manic by way of three cups of coffee and one impending free weights session, was that he had treated himself poorly; and worse, that he was involved in a zero-sum game, wherein he willingly sacrificed dignity to curry favor. He did not dispute my observations, though he was taken aback by how little wiggle-room I was interested in granting him, and the intensity with which I refused to grant it at the crack of dawn. He also asked, "Why do you care so much?" That was a good question. I certainly cared a lot. And so, I thought about it.

The truth is that at the time, I thought more than I did anything. It was a particular kind of thought, though. It wasn't about what I ought to do with my life or how exactly I went from studying political science in Virginia to working out obsessively and slinging calamari in New York. In fact, it wasn't really about me at all—or at least, to whatever extent obsessive thinking could ever be *not about the thinker*, it wasn't. All of my thought was aimed at existence, at purpose and meaning. Until that point in my life, there had always been some kind of template to be followed, as is the case for many people. Given my background, I always sort of knew that I would head to college after high school, that I would do something or another after that, and that eventually I'd be an adult—maybe even with a house, a yard, and some other people whom I'd tricked into living with me.

If that template I just offered seems riddled with gaps and lacking in detail, yes, it surely was. This was the problem. It translated into nothing real, which meant that at age 23, I found myself college-educated and waiting tables in New York, in a state of genuine and perpetual amazement that anyone could know precisely how they ought to operate in the world. How does anyone know? How does anyone *really know*? I was so drawn to this question of knowing. To say that it intrigued me would be the understatement of understatements. Eventually, it took the most extreme form it could: how does anyone *really know* anything? However paradoxical, my own waywardness seemed to trigger a question that compelled me like nothing had before.

Prior to then, I had not found much in the world I was particularly interested in, with one striking exception—baseball—but I noticed very quickly that I had more interest in these existential questions than nearly every single person I came across. Some people humored me. They would talk with me endlessly about seemingly unanswerable questions, the kind to which I slowly became more and more magnetized. Other people provided the simplest, most straightforward answers to really hard questions, as if there was nothing to think about—a strategy that obviously worked well-enough for them. Importantly though, I was quite open to whatever it was people thought about the issue at hand. Whether someone felt that biology or God destined all thought, feeling, and behavior; that personal choice ruled; or that everything in the world was wholly arbitrary, I listened. I listened, talked, and then thought. After that, I probably thought some more. I was preoccupied with huge questions but always more preoccupied with the methods by which people answered them.

Now, when you think of someone sifting through unanswerable questions, you assume that something like bias necessarily informs their answers. That is, if a question truly cannot be answered, yet someone has answered it nonetheless, it might be fair to assume that their answer reflects more about them than the question. I was able to suspend this truism to some degree, but not via virtue or skill. It just so happened that at this time in my life, I really and truly felt that nothing could be known, that no question could be legitimately answered (at least part of me did). You might say this is what I "knew." This meant, first, that I didn't have an obvious dog in any race, which I believe helped me see from many angles; and it meant, second, that my business wasn't so much answering questions as dismantling answers.

Admittedly, this made me a little difficult to be around at times, especially when one too many India Pale Ales did those in my surroundings the disservice of liberating me from my more natural, introverted state. At the drop of a hat, I would find the unspoken assumption in the other's belief system, then point out its flaws, assuming it had one—and it goes without saying, it always did. I had thought so much about these issues that I knew just where to push in order to poke an uncomfortable hole in a given worldview. This is not meant to aggrandize my thinking but to highlight my fixation. While most people were living their lives, concerned about the external world and the trajectory of their existences, I was obsessed with something much more hidden: the course by which "knowns" are arrived at.

Yet, despite my sense that things couldn't be known, I was secretly hoping that they could. This might be the best kept secret of every contemplative mind, but especially those still in development: a pervasive fantasy of absolute certitude. Thus, even while mounting (usually) friendly assaults on the givens and presuppositions held by others, I wanted desperately to understand why they held them. I wanted to know what could really be known, what was really true, and how it could be known to be true.

If someone wanted to argue that we know what we know, think what we think, and do what we do because of witchcraft, I would have listened. Ultimately, though, whether with self-proclaimed witches or anyone else, I never saw how people could separate what they *knew to be so* from what they *wanted to be so*. How could a half-thoughtful person really think that the knowns they generate from within and carry around with them were derived from objectivity or impartiality? I thought this was astoundingly shortsighted, so much so that when I encountered a person like this, I couldn't help but point out the outright bias and distortion contained in what their thoughts had returned to them (I might not have been the ideal dinner guest at this time in my life). However, owing to my skepticism about objectivity, I had no reason to think I knew anything definitively, either. How could I? I was fair about this, at least to the extent I could be. Strangely, I was full of openness to every possible idea as to how we might be able to know things, despite harboring sincere doubt that we could.

Regarding the whole enterprise of knowing, what I felt most certain of was just how little we could really know about our reasons for knowing what we do. I thought there were factors contributing to our conclusions—every possible variant, including opinions, inclinations, convictions—to which we simply lacked access, meaning we could never know about them. What's more, I thought we claim the validity of our pet ideas, never really knowing that their defining characteristic, the very thing that has made them appealing, is the fact that their shortcomings so happen to be of the variety that slide past our detection. This would mean that we systematically like ideas not for their validity but for the fault contained in them, to which we are blind, which is to say: we like ideas for the reasons we *cannot* see, not for the reasons we can. Nonetheless, when meant to explain how we arrived at a given idea or opinion, we faithfully track its development with no concern that there is anything else to know. But just how exactly would we know?

Moreover, what exactly does our reservoir of givens do for us? I thought about this idea for years, but to give the reader a sense of how preoccupied with it I truly was, I also lived it—or I wanted to. There were stretches of time where I tried to operate as if I had no givens. What I mean by no givens is no vested interest in anything, not an ounce of attachment to "outcome A" versus "outcome not A." I wanted to do this in order to see what life would be like, absent the assumptions we bring to it. Obviously, this is not possible to achieve fully, but it seemed so important to me that I tried. I'll just share one brief story to illustrate the point.

One weekend I aimed to wait tables as if I had no interest in how much money I made. I tried to deprogram my attachment to tips and thereby to my interest in gaining the favor and approval of customers, which, for waiters, is the taken-for-granted objective of every shift—every moment of every shift, even. This meant trying to drop all kinds of things that are taken as true, as supremely given. I wouldn't hurry per se if a table needed me, though I would not be rude either; I wouldn't small talk with customers if it wasn't a conversation I was truly interested in, but I also wouldn't behave dismissively; and I would always try to tell what I thought was the truth, whether or not it would earn me value in the eyes of the customer. If there is such a thing as waiter instincts, I had surely developed them, and I was now abandoning them. For example, if a waiter doesn't know much about wine (i.e., most waiters), one thing they like to do is to develop a kind of word bank of adjectives that subtly obscures their lack of expertise. And when used with confidence, they can choose nearly any of these words and accrue value to the customer for saying it. What is a "flowery finish" anyway? I still don't know.

On this weekend, I remember an exchange in which a very nice couple asked me for a recommendation. I told them I couldn't be fair because I didn't know wine that well, something I often said. But in this interaction, I took it closer to what was actually true for me: "Isn't it all the same? I tend to prefer bourbon to wine, and beer to bourbon, but I'm no expert in any of it." I also remember saying something like, "if we were a beer-only restaurant, you can be certain I'd be shooting my mouth off about my extensive beer knowledge." I was never rude, often self-deprecating, and always honest as I tried to drop my concern for outcomes—in this case, tips. After I said this, the couple decided to take advantage of our "bring your own" policy. They left the restaurant and returned five minutes later with a small bottle of bourbon. I was faced with a dilemma. Do I accept their invitation, have a seat at their table mid-shift, and share bourbon with them? Let me just come clean. It was no dilemma at all. I kindly accepted.

After all, what could be better proof that I had released all my pesky assumptions than being promptly fired? I'm kidding. Being fired wasn't in the cards; not only was the restaurant pretty empty but fraternizing with the customers might well have earned you employee of the month—this was the West Village.

Although this is a funny example, this whole enterprise—detaching from givens—was no joke to me. Not at all. I was deadly serious about rectifying what I took to be failures built into the process by which we "come to know." In doing so, I began to find unparalleled value in the questioning of my own assumptions, all of them. For a time, I considered the mere presence of my own opinions and inclinations, whether knee-jerk or well-thought-out, to be not simply harmful but completely immoral. As I saw it, in conviction—or conclusion of any kind—there could be no real truth, just real bias. To whatever extent it was possible, I wanted to eliminate my input. And because I was practicing detaching myself from certainty, this was easy for me, believe it or not; or at least, it was easier for me than for someone with immediate and natural trust that wherever their inkling has brought them is a place fashioned from outright legitimacy. This kind of person thinks, "I believe it; therefore, it is so!" I was the opposite. I had no such faith, which helped me to think and sometimes to be (e. g., drinking bourbon with friendly customers) in a rather odd way. While in this mode, however, I found that people were entirely unmotivated to join me. Assumptions are something people don't generally let go of so freely. This is true for many reasons, one of which follows obvious logic: we could not live without assumptions, and so we cannot really give them up. While this is true, it is not the truest reason for our death grip on all we hold to be so (a theme explored later).

Letting go of everything I thought I knew worked like a kind of faith at this time in my life. I was sure there was something important about it but didn't know what exactly. I also knew I couldn't achieve it fully and completely, and that a main obstruction was me and my identity—all I knew I was. This prompted an eruption of thought about what the self was and what function it was meant to serve. As I thought it through, I began to see personal knowledge as the primary and prized possession of the self—the very stuff of the self. This seemed important—that the self is defined by, more than anything else, what it has derived as so. To let go of what one takes to be true, in some very real and practical way, is to lose oneself, which also meant, though I hadn't recognized it yet, that it might well be the only route to lasting change. I became extraordinarily interested in ideas like these, but they were not maximally helpful to me yet because I couldn't see why I cared about them. I just did. They just were important; after all, for some reason or another, they had hijacked my mind, without apology.

So, there I was in New York, thinking obsessively about big questions. I was wondering what was knowable, if anything; whether we could ever really arrive at objective knowledge, given our involvement in knowing; and how any individual person could un-bias themselves from their own knowledge reserves in their pursuit to understand the world. I was also exercising fanatically, which was a surprisingly good forum for rumination. I thought and thought and thought—and I continued to talk about these things as well. Over time, I found people who were also curious about this stuff—and not in the places you'd necessarily expect. I preferred the brut, fearless, and at times aggressive thought of normal people to the refined, proper, and sanctioned thought of those who discuss philosophical matters as a means of being (or seeming) erudite. I had some experience waiting on the latter group both at cafes and restaurants, though they were never really for me (this is putting it lightly).

Eventually, I became extraordinarily close with my distant cousin, Sam, who is much older than me and had lived in New York for years. We spent many dinners sharing good food and introspection. Then, my brother and most trusted friend, Jamie, came to town. For a while before that though, my closest confidant was a "super" in the neighborhood, a maintenance man for an apartment around the corner from mine. We started chatting after seeing each other at a laundromat several times in the early afternoon, mid-week. Our first interaction? He points at a dryer full of women's underwear that had just finished its cycle and while making unbroken eye-contact with me, says, "I think your stuff is ready." In some strange way, it was as warm as it was hostile. Neither of us worked 9 to 5, and so we talked for a while that day. He was an ex-con, and he immediately became a friend.

He had done terrible things when he was young, all of which I eventually heard about in detail. He was such a human—so troubled, so troubled by being troubled, and so disarmingly honest about what he had done and why he thought he had done it. And so full of suffering. He had higher volumes only of insight than aggression. He was rough and cynical, but also hilarious and wise. One day while we smoked cigarettes on the stoop in front of his building, mere moments after informing me that I shouldn't be training for marathons and smoking simultaneously, he pointed out that for someone who thought knowing was impossible, I sure needed to know. What was this? A stoop intervention? I told him my therapist might want him to sign a no-compete. Yet, he was right to point out that something was amiss. This same thing had mystified me. I couldn't quite see why I was so concerned about these ideas. I was so steeped in thinking that thought was itself in the way of learning. Thought was in the way of knowing. And then, one day, it wasn't.

A Mystical Encounter

One Friday in November, I was walking from the subway station to the restaurant where I worked. I had not exercised that day for one reason or another, which at that time created a touch of angst. The streets were relatively empty given the usual hubbub of the West Village, but they were especially empty for a Friday. I was about two blocks from the restaurant. There was a guy walking toward me on the same side of the street, and another person, a woman, walking toward me on the other side. The trees lining the street were almost bare, though there were some brown leaves scattered throughout. It was dark too—it seemed more like 7 pm than 4 pm—and although it wasn't particularly cold, it was windy.

Suddenly, I was overwhelmed with the distinct sense that I was walking toward a restaurant that might or might not be there. It seemed like a ghost town. For a second, I thought it was one; and for a half-second, it was one. What were these people doing here? The man with whom I shared a sidewalk was now passing me. He seemed like a business type. I imagined that he was heading to happy hour somewhere. Who would he be drinking with though, if this place was abandoned? It flashed into my mind that he and I could probably drink beer together and laugh a lot. The woman on the other side of the street was not so put together. She was on her phone and outwardly angry but panged with sadness only millimeters below the surface. She stopped short of the restaurant, fumbled around her bag, then unlocked her apartment door and went inside. I had never seen her before, but she lived right down the street from where I worked. And just like that, the three of us no longer shared the sidewalk, the neighborhood, the city. We parted despite never really being together.

Upon going our separate ways, I experienced the most staggering sensation, one I had never accessed before; more accurately, though, one that had never before accessed me. It was the deepest, most penetrating calm, but it wasn't only that. It was calm tinged with despair, only the calm had a way of winning out. It was unshakable serenity insofar as it would not be rattled by its coexisting counterpart: suffering. It wasn't exactly "calmness" but an even more profound, "calm-despite-ness." It was so novel, so peculiar, so powerful. While I could never say why, I was seized in these moments—or better yet, invaded—by more understanding of "knowing" than I had amassed in all past moments combined. It was something like an enlightenment, a truly awesome moment of clarity. It wasn't that I had acquired more or new knowledge, but rather, knowledge of a different kind. Today, I look back at this strange experience with the sense that I learned more from it than I could ever capture with words. It was the beginning of something. Incidentally, five years later, I would complete a master's thesis on the plausibility of single awe-filled moments to transform worldviews and life courses, at times radically and permanently.

Now, I will try to put words to what I learned in that fraction of a second, in which I was overtaken by a feeling I can only describe as "peaceful dread." Of course, writing about what I learned has a kind of round-hole-square-peg quality to it, since it wasn't language that taught me. Nonetheless, what follows is my attempt to explain the extraordinary sensation that overwhelmed me on that ordinary day, on an ordinary sidewalk, in an ordinary neighborhood.

An Effort to Say the Unsayable

All that stood in the way of the restaurant I worked at *truly not being there* was a whole history of people developing convictions about how things ought to be—a whole history of people *knowing*. Over time, a set of givens made the West Village into a place with restaurants, colleges, all kinds of people, and over-priced tapas. All of this came into being, it materialized, on the back of discernment and knowing, resulting in my more or less pleasant walk to work, through a world supplied with form: sidewalks, people heading to happy hour, and well-maintained tree lines. On that day and in that moment, however, I experienced this scene as an outright fiction. It wasn't real to me; the *form* wasn't real to me.

But I wasn't psychotic and never have been (despite strange musings to come). I knew it was all there to be touched, seen, and heard. Yet, I was positively disconnected from the tangible and material scene around me and, somehow, more connected to the scene from which it sprang. I don't know the order in which they took place, or if they occurred simultaneously, but two things happened on that day. One, the given and real external world, the neighborhood, faded into nothingness, in turn seeming basically false; and two, my sense of personal subjectivity did the same. Words cheapen the experience, but in terms of language, these events put me "in touch with something underneath the given." And in being there, I learned something about human life. I learned that whatever we reflexively take experience to be is not what experience *truly is*. Instead, it is what we have *done to experience* by supplying it with ourselves—with our own personal assumptions and knowledge.

While it is easy to understand that Bleecker Street's physical form was determined by those who planned and built it, this isn't really the point. My concern is not with the assumptions of city planners in downtown New York, or, frankly, with the physical world at all. On the contrary, what matters is that this model not only *holds* when applied to human subjectivity; it *accounts for* the nature of human subjectivity. The subjective experience we take as true, valid, real—comprised by our internal sidewalks and tree-lines—is always and eternally embedded in some very personal sense as to how things "ought" to be seen, just as the properties of the West Village required "oughts" to come into existence. There is a kind of desire threaded into subjectivity, always. In all my obsessive thinking, I had played with this idea before, but on this day, it wasn't an idea. It was an encounter. It shook me out of something, or into something. The strangest part of these very strange moments was the unusual effortlessness with which I saw the possibility of another, more primordial world, a world that pre-exists the one in which we find ourselves, the one we have littered with our input, assumptions, convictions, and knowledge. I suddenly knew, with a stunning ease, that the world we see is not the world; the world we see is the world as we wish to see it.

After that, my understanding of reality began to change, often in abrupt, choppy, and dramatic ways, since something foundational, I think within myself, was being reconstituted. With this eerie walk to work, knowledge began to mean something very different to me than what it had meant before. It shifted from a thing *we have* to a thing *we do*; and I slowly began to see that, regardless of its content, we all do it for the same reason. Each of us develops firm ideas, convictions, and beliefs about human experience as a means of keeping at arms-length one of its underlying yet ever-present elements, which would show itself all the time, if not for our protective, elaborate narratives. In suspending one's own input as to what human experience is, one might find (or be found by) a windy and dark ghost town, one lacking completely in form, yet somehow filled to its brim with loss.

Through inhabiting this world, I had just seen into a formula, which (I think) remains a secret to whatever extent a person trusts the processes and output of their own mind. In other words, when unshakable faith is attached to one's own perception, thought, and conclusions, one is fooled into seeing the given world— the one given to us by simple observation—as the realest world. I lacked such faith, or maybe I rejected it; whatever the case, doing so helped me—even caused me—to see some quite different things. On that day, I found a piece of knowledge that, for one reason or another, I could not dispute. I couldn't fight it with words; I couldn't argue it with reasons. It just was. The realm of being *just was* one of suffering, and the whole enterprise of perception *just was* an endogenous analgesic. So many operations of the human mind that I formerly took to be reality-finding in their function were, now, anything but. They were pain-relieving.

Aftershocks

After this experience, my mind broke open like a dam. I saw old questions, those about "knowing," from new angles. Specifically, if suffering really is an inescapable feature of being, then how could it not inform the "knowns" any person arrives at? But more to the point, how could our knowns not be dictated by it? I began to think that because it is so central to human life, what any of us consciously knows must be beholden to suffering; and further, that even if we are not exactly aware of how suffering informs our consciously held knowns, it still must. Here is a parallel. As we navigate the physical world, assuming we have not fallen off a cliff or landed on our heads, all of our conscious choices have taken account of underlying physical laws, like that of gravity. While we aren't required to know about these laws explicitly, nor are they part of our conscious calculus, all of our behavior models itself in a way that is wholly adherent to them. I was beginning to think the human mind worked in the same way: that all of our conscious mental behavior, from top to bottom, from start to finish, was somehow fueled by the underlying law of suffering.

My ideas about "knowing" then became more complicated—in a good way. Maybe people who were "certain," "positive," and "sure" were not simply corrupted or dysfunctional, unaware of their own mind's desirous aims; maybe knowing was fundamentally all about *need*. Maybe it wasn't such a problem that *what we know to be so* cannot be untied *from what we want to be so*. Maybe this was an inevitability. Suddenly I became much less concerned with whether knowing was really possible, or whether what we know could ever be considered "true." Instead, I found myself fascinated by the possibility that "knowing"—and all of the mind processes preceding it—was the most powerful tool we had in delivering ourselves from suffering. For so long, I had been asking *how* people can claim to know what they know, but this question, one about validity, now seemed ill-suited as a tool for understanding human experience; as I now saw things, it was far more important to ask *why* people have come to know what they know, a question whose answer, for all of us, includes suffering. This perspective, however, was not itself any final answer. It was only the beginnings of a good question.

From there, my preoccupations and my way of being in the world began to reroute themselves. I no longer oriented to knowns—mine or anyone else's—with unrelenting skepticism but with genuine respect because I had become convinced of their protective qualities. I had finally found something important about knowing. I only found it, though, without my doing, without my will whatsoever, on an average day in which I wasn't trying to do anything except walk to work and fake expertise about wine. I now thought that *maybe* our knowledge was verifiable and *maybe* it wasn't, but this question no longer moved me. I had graduated. What I now cared about was its status as *anything but arbitrary*. Somehow, knowledge was protective—*all of it*.

Yet this posed another, even bigger problem. How could we ever know new things, where knowing means holding real and true intrinsic conviction, if our existing knowledge somehow spares us pain and suffering? Why would anyone ever let go of what they know? For example, how could Vince come to *really know* that he is not mandated to treat himself poorly, even if doing so helps him in one way or another to minimize his own suffering, which from my new worldview, it necessarily did. This is a question about change, one we all must answer for ourselves, not just as psychologists but as people. The answer I have come to, began to come to me on a windy day in New York City in what feels like another life.

A Different World

I share this story because it marks a significant change in my life. Following this series of events, I began to think very differently about the world than I had in the past. But it wasn't just a change in thought. It was more fundamental than that. My perception had changed, and I knew it. I was actually seeing differently; it was as if my eyes were working in a way they had not before. The world around me had changed, even though I also knew it hadn't. It was something internal that shifted. I want to quickly assure the reader that, as a person, my concerns are with reality and truth, and so while some of what I am offering might sound flimsy and sentimental, please bear with me. I would acknowledge that what I am saying is strange, but it is not overdramatized or fanciful (and I hope to further convince you of this throughout the book).

I soon realized that whatever I was previously, I wasn't any more. It's odd and sadly cliched to say it this way, but sometimes phrases endure because they capture something true: I really had endured a kind of death and rebirth. But what to do with this new life? Well, I knew that it involved understanding. While I had always been interested in understanding the human mind, I was all at once inspired to be *understanding of* the human mind. Somehow, a goal of appreciating human life, especially its inbuilt problems, had simply found me. I wanted to make more sense of suffering because I was sure there was a path to alleviating it, and I was also sure each of us was our own best hope; or that through our own internal capacities, we were at least a central part of the solution. I had become terribly interested in how people might change subjectivity for the better. Yet, this was not a primarily intellectual or philosophical pursuit. Ideas were not the draw. People were. I wanted to know how we as human beings could find more peace despite the state in which we find ourselves—content, but not forever; connected, but not forever; safe, but not forever; *alive, but not forever.*

Back to Thinking

Before I returned to school for a PhD in clinical psychology, I spent more time wondering about what I thought about human improvement: how exactly do people get better, psychologically speaking, and what is the role of the other in the process? I was pretty sure I had an idea of what the academic world thought about these questions. Despite having very little interest in learning while in college, I managed to pick up the idea that biological predispositions, socio-cultural factors, and idiosyncratic psychological factors (i.e., the "biopsychosocial model") were behind one's way of being in the world. However, by the time I became personally interested in the mind, I could not see how biological, psychological, or social processes had much to do with the alleviation of suffering, *even if each of them had a role in creating it.* It wasn't exactly that I disagreed that the nature of someone's suffering is multidetermined or that their history is relevant to the here-and-now. I understood all of this; what I didn't understand was why all of it necessarily mattered to healing.

I just couldn't see how models like these (e.g., biopsychosocial) were germane to a psychotherapeutic encounter. Back then, before I was actually sanctioned to sit across from a suffering person, I imagined doing so. What would I do in that moment based on his or her biopsychosocial precursors? Might I tweak their temperamental endowments (bio), alter their attachment history (psycho), or revise the cultural milieu in which they happened to grow up (social)? And if these were my goals, how would I achieve them with my words? I was considering becoming a psychologist, not a genie, which meant these routes wouldn't work—not in the absence of either a time machine or delusions of grandeur. When it came to change, I always wondered, what is the meaning of *this moment* and what are *this moment's* tools?

As I spent more and more time with this problem, my thinking became more and more radical compared with the standards of academic psychology. Of course, I knew very little about academic psychology at the time I started in on these problems, which was well before I returned to school for a PhD or even considered doing so. I had begun thinking through these matters without having yet learned anything from the most learned, and I was hovering around the idea that a person's history wasn't as important in the actual therapeutic encounter—in the mechanisms of healing—as might be assumed. The obedient, rule-following practitioner has probably never earnestly questioned whether a person's past has relevance to the therapeutic encounter. They assume it does; then they know it does because they are taught it does. I was not nearly as agreeable to the conventional wisdom, but not as a result of mere rebelliousness. I knew that a person's way of being in the world, including the nature of their pain, suffering, and hardship, was produced by thousands of unknowable variables, including historical ones; I just couldn't see how this information was of primary value in the therapy room.

Even while training in academic psychology and flying under the radar as something like an existentialist with a soul (with the protection of beloved advisers), I accepted all the scientific "knowns" of human development: neurological, interpersonal, sociological, etc. What we have learned through science about how people develop is not at all *wrong*, nor was I worried about the extent to which it was *accurate*. I was worried about the extent to which it was useful to the person sitting across from me. I wanted to cut through all the abstracted, empirically sanctioned knowns (i.e., psychological and psychotherapeutic models and facts) and understand the role of each passing moment. I wanted to know, "what is the meaning of the therapeutic encounter itself?"

I devoted almost all of my thought to this question well before I was authorized by the academic establishment to think at all. I do not say this to disparage academia or the powers that be in clinical psychology. I say it to make clear to the reader that I am not really writing this book as a psychologist, even though I am one, but as a thinking person who started thinking about these issues prior to learning anything about the rules of the game. Lucky for me, graduate school provided more time to think, now with other people, about the nature of both suffering and its alleviation. Throughout, I returned time and time again to the meaning of a person's "knowns."

At the time, I would often run myself (and others) through thought experiments like this one. Imagine two people. First, a hypervigilant young man, who stealthily carries a pocket-knife in an extremely low-crime neighborhood for fear that he will be attacked; second, another young man of the same age, who seeks out high-crime areas precisely so he can carry around religious pamphlets and attempt to embrace (and convert) anyone who crosses his path. Obviously, these people are different in countless ways and have become different for countless reasons. Even so, couldn't we say that *right now*—in the moment one is preparing to fight, and the other is preparing to preach—the factor that most distinguishes the conscious life of one from the conscious life of the other is the knowns by which it is populated? They know extraordinarily different things about themselves, others, and the world, don't they? This means something about change. It must. It has to.

If we could do one thing to improve the psychological health of the first man above, what would it be? Anyone whose answer to that question takes the form of a *thing* from the external world (e.g., give him a brand-new house!) will not like much of this book. For those still reading, let's try to keep things purely psychological, here. My answer always went something like this: if I could wave some magical wand and do one thing to help someone struggling to exist in their own psyche, I would give them new knowns. They would suddenly just *know new things*. For the first guy above, imagine how much his life would change if he abruptly knew that other people are not made of unprovoked malice, nor are they even particularly interested in him. This new knowledge would take care of much of his strife, wouldn't it? I thought so.

With this, my view of the relationship between suffering and knowing was becoming even more complicated. Even if our knowns protected us from a certain amount of pain, which I thought they surely did, somehow, they also held great potential to spawn just as much of it. I was becoming more certain that where people have landed in their minds—their givens, axioms, and assumptions—held *actual* power to *actually* destroy them, full stop. In turn, I found what I thought mattered and could be helpful in moment-to-moment experience with people—a kind of guiding principle, not just for therapy but for human suffering and its alleviation. If people are to live with less agony, could it be that they simply need to *know different things?*

You might find that this sounds too narrow, simplistic, or weighted toward cognition to be considered a viable path to change. But it's none of these things. Let me explain. First of all, it is not my intention to dismiss every proven origin of "pathological experience," including those uncovered in empirical studies having to do with genes, history, and environment. My intention is only to pose that despite its origins, the most immediate problem for someone tortured by a hellish first-person experience—immediate in their waking life—is found in what they take, axiomatically, as so. The power of this idea is seen when you consider replacing one person's givens with those of another person. What would change? My guess was the entirety of their experience would. That is, *what we know* and *how we experience* are very tightly related.

In a way, this is the assumption that grew this whole book, every thought that went into it, and more frankly, the whole course of my adult life. Call to mind any person who has struggled with existence, any person plagued by the nature of their own subjectivity, and ask this very simple question: could you ever separate the misery of their life from the givens of their mind? A suffering person has taken things as so that cause them harm (this can be said with no assertions as to whether what they know is "true"). In turn, if these things could be revised, if other things could be taken as so, perhaps life could be quite different. Simply put, if a person can know things anew, the world might present itself in a very different way.

Maybe I sound to the reader like a good old-fashioned cognitivist, a group openly in the business of changing knowns (i.e., think this, not that!). But let me assure you, I am not that, nor have I ever been that, not even when my ideas were first developing. I just didn't think people worked like that. I agreed with the cognitivists that we want people to know different things in *their* minds, but I could not believe for the life of me that the path to doing so was to confront them with *ours*. It's too easy, too simplistic. You can't just make someone know different things because you think they "should," whatever your reasons. I thought people who see it this way must overvalue cognition at the very least and probably their own influence as well. I had never met anyone who changed their mind by being *taught* that they should, including myself—actually, *especially* myself. This put me in a bind. I was no cognitivist as my own experience ruled it out.

But it also put me on a path. Understanding the meaning and development of a person's knowledge became synonymous, for me, with understanding their life, its problems, and maybe even the path to change. Could knowing new things yield a new reality? I thought the crudest answer was yes, but I still didn't have a great handle on how it would work. I just knew I was relentlessly skeptical of psychology's beloved cognitive-behavioral therapy (CBT), the cognitive piece of which teaches people why they ought to acquire new knowns and precisely how to do so. CBT assumes one person can willfully and readily intervene into the cognition of another and make an adjustment or two where necessary. While this is surely a useful ethos for tailors working on inseams, it was less clear to me that we therapists can (or should) aim for that same level of power over another's mind.

Yet, *I did think* people needed to think differently. I just didn't know how, in part because I wasn't so sure about what our knowns—our knowledge—meant to begin with. What was it? Was it revisable? Could another person revise it? I didn't know, but I wanted to. I wanted to better understand the meaning of knowledge. Crucial to the story is that I wanted to orient to "knowledge" with a complete and wholesale disregard for the knowledge designations that we, modern man, have provided ourselves (e.g., fact, opinion, wisdom). I wasn't interested in these categories, but not because I took them as false. In some sense, they captured true distinctions. Rather, because as I saw it, there must have been a point at which human minds had created them. And in this sense, each category, however different in kind, was produced by the same phenomenon, which is native to the human mind; namely, the process by which it arrives.

Whether fact or belief, folk-knowledge or empirical data, in order to have arrived at it and accepted it as "so," the mind of the arriver had to have gotten there. It had to have been, at the very least, involved. To be clear, I didn't think all knowledge was equally valid (and incidentally, I'm no radical postmodernist). I did think, however, that anything people claim to know had to have been, in some genuine sense, *believed in*, whether it would be characterized with words as opinion, fact, or nonsense. How do we arrive at things, period, was my question, whether at the idea that our neighbor is short-tempered, that the ice-caps are melting, or that one religion is superior.

I wanted to take a 300,000-foot view of the process by which the human mind concludes, lands, or forecloses. I would often imagine being dropped into the world at several different points in history, and just told "Go!" What would I take to be "given" in different eras? Are today's facts yesterday's facts; are today's convictions tomorrow's convictions? And most importantly, how do ever-changing givens impact subjective experience? That is, how are the qualities of one's conscious knowns and the qualities of one's consciousness related? I also wondered how it happened that, since the times of the earliest people, we have made so many demarcations around "so-ness." For example, X is a fact, but Y is opinion, and Z is really a crazy idea altogether. How does the human mind make certain things more valid than others? Or is validity somehow bestowed by the external world, only to be apprehended or perceived by each of us? In essence, I was interested in how the mind has come to take as so what the mind now takes as so, whatever it might be, however it might be characterized.

Knowing is Alive

Ultimately, this period in my life taught me what knowledge isn't. It isn't static, abstracted, or inert; and, of special importance, it isn't something that could ever possibly be partitioned from the knower. To the contrary, it is alive in every moment of each person's subjective experience—and this is the meaning of the therapeutic encounter: to find it operating *right now*, and somehow intervene, in order to set it on a different course. The question, of course, is how.

Throughout all of my thinking, laid out above, I was really searching for answers to three related questions: 1) why do people know what they know; 2) how can knowns be altered; and 3) what is the role of another person (i.e., a psychologist) in altering them? As I delved deeper into these very cerebral and intellectual questions—all of those I had about the nature, meaning, development, and revision of "knowns"—they eventually gave way to answers that were nothing of the sort. The only explanations that satisfied me, even remotely, turned out to be preposterously simple. These same questions, which I took so seriously as to test the limits of my own sanity, began to yield answers *so modest* as to seem patently and almost unbelievably absurd. I say that genuinely. I didn't believe myself at first, but nor could I see any way out of it—and nor have

I since. After years of dedicated, endless, and at times unwanted thinking, as well as chronic grappling with the nature of myself but also the nature of human experience in general, I was finally able to find answers to the three questions above. The very last step in doing so, inspired by that strange encounter on a New York City sidewalk, was to see that despite having formulated three questions—and despite the human tendency to formulate questions, whatsoever—to these questions and all others, there has only ever been one consistently viable answer. The simplest and best answer is love.

From time to time, I still think about Vince, my friend from the café, though I haven't talked with him in years. What I hope is that he has been able to revise his knowns—that he now knows he doesn't have to treat himself badly. But if he has come to really and truly know new things, it is very unlikely he got there by way of thought, for changes in mind are not simply changes in mind. Knowing is a matter of things infinitely deeper than that.

AN INTRODUCTION TO THE BOOK'S BROADEST PURPOSES

This book's most specific goal is to convey a message to the field of clinical psychology about what psychotherapy is, what it isn't, and how we ought to think about it. As illustrated in the Preface, these are questions to which I have given significant thought. However, because my view of the therapeutic encounter is ultimately only my view of human experience, adjusted for a particular interpersonal situation we call "psychotherapy," there is another sense in which I've given these questions very little directed thought, at all. That is, only after first thinking fanatically about human transformation, did I have a single thought about its implications for professional psychology. For this, there are implications important to this book, which I want to admit to the reader, here.

I have a view of human life before I have a view of "clinical work;" a view of human relationships before a view of a "therapeutic relationship;" a view of a helpful person before a view of a "therapist;" and a view of the nature of suffering before a view of "psychopathology." Throughout this book, then, any time I am talking about my understanding of "clinical work" or "patients," I'm only half-talking about these things as we currently think of them; more fundamentally, I'm talking about my understanding of *relationships* and *people*, which are contemporarily dubbed "clinical work" and "patients," respectively, when they happen to be situated behind certain doors. The point here is that my view of clinical work couldn't possibly be separated from my view of everything else. They are one and the same.

All of this is important for the reader to know because it matters with respect to this book's purposes. I do in fact want to influence how my field thinks about itself. This is true. At the heart of it, though, my perspective about the nature of clinical work is, so too, a perspective about the nature of human experience. And

DOI: 10.4324/9781003305286-1

so, the real target of this book lies past not only the field of clinical psychology but past institutions altogether. This will become evident as the text progresses, but the deepest point I am trying to make is one about *what people* are, which has implications not only for how "therapists" ought to treat "patients" but for how persons ought to treat each other.

I want to use the current section to introduce the book by way of its most recurrent paths of thought, which manifest continuously and throughout. In one way or another, they show themselves in every section, even in every word, perhaps unsurprisingly so, since they reflect the author's deepest-seated sensibilities. Regardless of what I am writing about, psychotherapy or life, or how I am writing about it, with indignance, humor, or sympathy, there are a couple of things I am always trying to achieve. These might be thought of as the book's most prominent through lines; they are the through lines of intention, and there are two. The remainder of this section will first lay them out, and in doing so, give way to an introduction to this book's most central proposition.

Intention One: Toward Self-Reflection and Thinking

This book's first intention is to foster thought. I want everyone to think more. I understand that most people reading this book are already interested in thinking and already very good thinkers. So, I don't mean this pedantically as in, "I'll teach you how to think," nor do I mean it egoistically as in, "I'll show you why you should think more *like me*." Of course, some will take to what I lay out; others will reject it; others will do some of both. Fair enough. My hope is not that everyone agrees with this text but that everyone who journeys through it will contend with what I offer, thereby firming up their own ideas at the very least; and at the very most, finding within themselves more independence of thought— *more of themselves.*

We all need to know what we think, what we really think, especially those of us alleging to have some value to people who are suffering. This is truer for clinicians and therapists than for any other healthcare professional. Think of it. While your gastroenterologist was training and developing expertise, their instincts as to the innerworkings of the stomach mattered very little. The stomach works how it works; and for the good of their future patients, medical doctors in-training would be well served to drop most of their creative, artistic, or intuitive instincts about its processes. Some in psychology conceptualize psychic problems in the same way: "this is what depression is, this is how it works, and this is how you fix it." Unfortunately, this view is thoughtless at best. Talk with a person for 15 minutes and any remaining attachment to a-priori ideas about how their suffering "ought" to be treated indicates only a lack of curiosity or creative thought. This is why all therapists should try to lay out—at least in their minds, if not in a book—precisely what they think and why. We are charged with improving the subjectivity of other people. If this doesn't prompt significant reflection and unending thought, what could?

Reflection is for Everyone

Yet, my goal of promoting reflection, like this book in general, is not meant for clinicians only. Reflection is for everyone. Unfortunately, in the modern world, it is a capacity in which *everyone* is also rapidly losing both skill and interest. What's worse, those who have managed to retain it are certainly not rewarded for having done so—quite the opposite, actually. While it is probably true that the conditions of contemporary life—being saturated in technology, surrounded by opportunities for immediate gratification, and encouraged to do everything faster—have contributed to its development, we human beings are now stuck with a problem, however it came about. We are nearly allergic to real and genuine introspection. What's more, this allergy is now built right into the things we build, which means *we* have no chance to build any tolerance against *it*.

Before delving too much further into what I hope is a fair critique of modern life, I need to say something very explicitly to the reader. I am certainly critical of much that surrounds us in 2022. There is no doubt about this. But there is also good reason for it. I see human beings as agents of self-transformation, capable of unknown potential for growth, endowed with a natural instinct to revise—if not abolish—every previously held idea that has obstructed them on the path to ethical and spiritual betterment. It is precisely a scarcely containable faith in the human spirit—its capacities for reflection, self-understanding, goodwill, and psychic triumph of all kinds—that causes modern life to look like the opening act of a tragedy. People can—and must—be victors in the struggle with their own psyches, but doing so requires time spent with oneself and with one's own innerworkings. This is not a pursuit that modern values merely "discourage." We should be plain and truthful. It is a pursuit that modern values burn to the ground.

This is a problem for individual persons because the instinct to transformation, like any other instinct, can be thwarted in the wrong environment. That wrong environment is 2022. I count myself lucky insofar as I became, for lack of a better word, *obsessed* with internal life and psychic change as a young person. But short of being naturally preoccupied with these issues, I'm not sure how anyone would develop even a slight taste for them, given our current situation. Those whose natural instinct to see themselves truthfully is somewhat muted will not be pushed by modern culture to further draw it out, grow it, and live in accordance with it. In turn, they will gain little perspective on themselves or the world around them, causing them to find few problems with life as it now stands. Our rampant utilitarianism, our obsession with productivity and efficiency, nor the empty nihilism these values foster will cause them any worry.

Such people are often characterized as naïve, and they are, but being naive does not preclude one from being hazardous (only unbridled sentimentalism would lead to that conclusion). Lacking the discernment to see that business as usual is corrupt, they accept the status quo, so too accepting, in effect, the assault on the human spirit embedded within it—even if unwittingly. As they are unable to see and assess decay, nor can they notice when there is something to be restored, which quietly (but firmly) obviates any need for hope, and thereby any relationship with it. While self-reported cynics are without hope because they cannot muster it, unwitting cynics (formerly, "the naïve") are without hope because they see no utility for it. The traditional cynic says, "Human integrity is a pipedream. *This* is just how it is." The unwitting cynic I am proposing here says, "What do you mean there's something wrong with *this*? Might there be something wrong with *you*?" Effectively, both believe that "there is nothing to see here." Both are wrong.

The latter is a more special case of cynicism, though, because it is blind to itself. One who cannot see problems fails also to see that critique, for which they have an aversion, is actually born of the very hope that their blindness makes unnecessary. They even mistakenly fancy themselves optimists. But optimism in someone who sees nothing wrong is not real optimism, just as an apology given by someone who feels no guilt is not a real apology. It's only empty optimism. What these strange cynics mean to say is that the sound of critical thought hurts their ears, and the sight of scrutiny, their eyes. It is this trait—not brave acceptance, not hard-won self-transcendence, and certainly not genuine optimism—that allows them to scan the world, wholly unperturbed. It's also the reason they wish you would too, for exposure to all your contemplation as to what's *really going on* is peeling the rose-tint from their glasses and the unearned serenity from their minds. There is little virtue in this orientation. It's destructive and cynical—and the fact that it is these things *unknowingly* couldn't possibly make it these things *any less*. My intent is not to be harsh toward this kind of person; but rather, to point out that the false optimism afforded by blindness and the apathy of plain old cynicism are functionally the same—and equally misguided.

Unfortunately, the nature of modern society makes it challenging for either group to see the error of their ways. Why? Because errors are only *necessarily* seen when they are seen internally. Traditional cynics will change not when they find virtue and nobility in the world but when they find both in themselves; likewise, the traditionally naïve will not change when they finally see darker forces in the world *around them* but in the world *within them*. Unfortunately, both outcomes are unlikely in our world because incentives to earnestly introspect, seriously question, and see oneself from new angles are nowhere to be found.

Reflection? Not on 2022's Watch

First of all, most people are so busy that they don't have time to look up, let alone look inward. With what exactly have they busied themselves? Many things, all of which converge on the *pursuit of more*. By this, I do mean the usual culprits—more money, more toys, and a second beach house—all of which are attained through a wholly external orientation (i.e., in order to get the material goods, one must get out into the stuff-filled world and claim what's theirs!). But we are also *pursuing more* in a way that is much deeper and more harmful to us. We are after excess not only in the material world but in our internal worlds. All of modern life's comfort and control has given us the wrong impression of what subjective experience is. Namely, we take ourselves as its high ruler; as such, we command things from it. We believe it should contain certain things and not others. To many in the modern world, subjective experience will do only when it is free of strife and filled with ease; lacking in grief and abundant in joy; and devoid of limitation and brimming with potential. When one finally manages to strip their self-deception of any governor whatsoever, one arrives at the most damning notion of all: one's own permanence.

After only a bit of thought, we already see something strange here, don't we? Our material aims, all we chase after in the external world (e.g., soon-to-be-obsolete gadgets, new cars, and that third beach house), have a not-so-hidden psychological function. They have a hand in keeping us away from ourselves, away from our internal lives. Setting one's sights on all the (false) treats of the external world and then furiously gathering them up is a perfect way to avoid oneself. Doing so not only undermines any relationship one might build with themselves; it can even stamp out one's awareness of one's own subjectivity, entirely. Think of how unholy this alliance really is. In successfully acting out modern society's highest value (i.e., collecting maximal *stuff*), one all but inoculates themselves from reflection, which is to say, one all but inoculates themselves from themselves. At that point, the pursuit of reflection loses any and all value it might otherwise have because, according to prevailing standards, it isn't worth much. Technically speaking, it isn't worth anything. After all, you can't pay for your next I-phone with self-awareness, can you? In an alternative world, one in which people were frothing at the mouth over "the next upgrade" in self-understanding, society would boast a slightly better chance of not running headlong off a cliff.

What we have, then, is an entire society that, as a system, is itself motivated to keep people away from genuine reflection, and for a very simple reason: the frenetic hunt for stuff and comforts (our stated reason for existing), does not require of us any internality. In turn, our capacity for looking within atrophies. Eventually, when the majority of people comprising society are unable to reflect or think very deeply at all because all of their energy and attention is aimed exclusively outward, society has to change. It must remake itself in accordance with—that is, it must accommodate—the psyche of its citizenry. What does this look like? It looks like the reinforcing and strengthening of every psychological impulse that came to obstruct us from reflection in the first place. And it's already happened.

Ask yourself: is it a coincidence that the world no longer asks of people things like patience, prudence, or the ability to delay pleasure? Of course, it isn't. The creators of everything valuable enough to be called an "advance" wouldn't dream of requiring these things of us; if they did, their product could never develop a sufficient consumer base to be considered an advancement. Just imagine a new game for your phone being marketed for the significant time commitment and critical thought it requires. It would fail to sell because a game like this is hardly the fix for someone's 12-minute train ride to work, in which they seem determined to forget they exist (and thanks to Facebook and other apps, often do so at a disturbing rate of success). When looked at in this way, our situation is nothing short of perverse. The things we most value are the things that most alienate us from ourselves. But don't tell us that—we would surely object, with a fist in the air (provided we've mastered one-handed texting).

Our situation is one in which the world's most powerful technologies are being unwittingly used to destroy the inner lives of its own citizens, all of whom are strangely complicit. That is, for those to whom they are marketed, society's advances seem quite helpful, which is the singular goal of marketing and the reason we accept them as if they are wine and not poison. After all, our "technological progress" often comes to us in tasty and otherwise appealing packages, doesn't it? Want to be eating a pizza in less than eight minutes? Want a girlfriend? A new boyfriend? A better pizza? A better girlfriend? The "perfect pizza?" Want a fanbase for any fleeting idea? Piece of cake (by the way, want a piece of cake?). All of this—and much, much more—can be yours in the modern world.

But what exactly are we doing to people as we blur—or worse, eradicate once and for all—the line between fantasizing and having? What have we done to people when they walk around the world believing that something has gone wrong if gratification fails to be the baseline state of subjectivity? We have further devastated the possibility that anyone will ever go inward and stay a while. Modern life puts people on a never-ending quest for something better, a quest invariably aimed outward, which means not just that we will remain unfamiliar with ourselves; we will also be made into creatures of reaction, impulse, and pleasure. In being driven toward the cheapest sources of thrill by the most surface aspects of ourselves, we become less human. This is the path we are on, whether or not all of us can open our eyes to it—and many simply cannot because who bites the hand that feeds you wines and cakes and illusions?

Non-Reflection Means Disconnection from Self and Other

Non-reflection first means disconnection from ourselves. Just look around. We know nothing of entertainment that isn't primarily distracting, and we like everything we like precisely for its ability to pull us away from ourselves and into an escapist world of illusion. Unfortunately, we have lost ourselves in not only matters of fun and play but in matters of human purpose (the former of which turn out to be critical to a good life but mean nothing in the absence of the latter). These days, clubs and groups exist precisely for their ability to pad a resumé or to catapult a budding person into the right college and thereby a more respectable, less detestable status (detestable to them and anyone else who equates a meaningful title with a meaningful life). Is achievement striving a problem? No, not in itself; but instrumentally joining something for its promise to yield standing is a far cry from joining something because it speaks to one's heart and mind. Unfortunately, because society is facilitating the destruction of introspection, many people are unable to make this distinction. They genuinely can't.

In being distant from ourselves, our naturally affinity for contending with multiple aspects of ourselves is degraded, which worsens our ability to contend with multiple aspects of others—or even *one* aspect of them we don't like. This is why contemporary work life requires a paid babysitter's club, called "Human Resources"—so that full-grown adults, instead of *reflecting* on their contribution to some petty conflict and working it out with their difficult co-worker, can have the option of engaging in unvarnished egoism, all while maintaining their sense of justified outrage. Just picture someone storming into a room labeled "HR" and throwing the richest temper-tantrum you can imagine, one with all the trappings: disavowal of responsibility, maligning the other person completely, and maybe even a little foot-stomping for good measure. It wouldn't be wise to betray any sense of responsibility or remorse in the presence of HR; after all, the modern world shows us that its real players apologize for nothing. In fact, according to contemporary life, one must stand righteously for one's own rights before standing at all for one's responsibilities to others.

This phenomenon is perhaps most clearly seen on the little slice of hell known as social media. What happens to communication and discourse when the people attempting to engage in it are unable to think critically about much of anything, including their own motivation? "Twitter" does. Not only does this platform not require the human virtues of reflection, critical thought, or mutual respect; it all but exiles them. Think of how strange this is: a platform holding itself out as a place for discourse relies on the absence of an attention span in its user. As it allows only 140 characters, in order to be admitted, one must curb their thought as a cover charge. Who knows? Maybe this number, 140, was yielded by focus groups that proved 141 would be bad for business. One could argue, "But Rob, people don't *really* go there for discourse." Maybe you don't think so, but the people who go there certainly do. And there aren't many good alternatives, either. Apart from longform podcasts, all public discourse has the same problem. It is constituted by an "exchange of ideas" that is nothing more than primitive reactions and impulses ping-ponging back and forth, only veiled in words. People engage to tell, not to listen; to assault, not to learn; to win, not to collaborate. Thoughtful dialogue isn't exactly a strength of ours, and Twitter, whatever its representatives say, doesn't want it to be.

Sadly, to gain competency in dialogue as modern life defines it, one must only harness triteness and glibness; and to see prevailing standards of communication as deficient, one would have to maintain the ability to reflect and see oneself clearly, which happens to be the very skill Twitter discourages. In order to make discernments about the nature of the contribution one is putting forth, including its depth, importance, and complexity, one must be able to reflect. One must be able to go into oneself and ask what is behind one's own offering. And what might be? Well, anything might be, but a person's ability to grasp what's *really* there—what *really* motivates them—is limited by their potential for self-reflection. If their potential is close to zero, all of their "tweets," all of their convictions in general, might be driven by everything other than what they claim them to be. A sense of injury, elitism, righteousness, or blind and sentimental loyalty might well move one to say what they did, despite their claim that it grew from the very springs of contemplation, consideration, and fairness. This, a lack of self-reflection, is how people discharge incoherence and spite, all the while convinced that they are having a thoughtful, worthwhile exchange.

Not restricted to the false world of social media, this phenomenon now shows itself in more and more living rooms, around more and more kitchen tables, and within more and more workplaces. Real dialogue between any two people is meaningless if the parties involved cannot really reflect. Unfortunately, our society is not for reflection. The real consideration of ourselves? "No thanks," we say, as we snap yet another picture-perfect raspberry tart and frantically "post" it for all the world to see. We might be losing any sense as to who we are, but in due time our desserts will be regarded as superlative by every person we will never meet. I guess every society needs priorities.

Non-Reflection Compromises Independence of Thought

What I have always wanted is for people to rebel against *all they don't really know,* which is a category much larger than anyone is willing to admit. I take doubt as an uncelebrated virtue, not only because it makes people wise but because it makes people good. In today's world, however, this is a big ask. With every new day, we are increasingly certain of just exactly what the world is; with every new sunrise, there is less and less room to consider what else might be. Society is a colossally powerful machine that has added more than meets the eye—more than unthinkable skyscrapers, medical procedures, and technological advances. Modern life has also added psychological givens: there are things that are good and things that are bad, ideas that are smart and ideas that are dumb, perspectives that are kind and perspectives that are mean. Unfortunately, anyone who has not developed the capacity for self-reflection will not only depend on these givens; they will revere them.

Such reverence is dangerous though because it is an unwitting stance against oneself. Independent thought is only really available to people who have some idea of how they *really* feel about things, some idea of who they *really* are. Being an independent thinker starts with being an independent soul, which is facilitated not by the ability to think in an IQ sort of way; rather, it is facilitated by an ability to make a home in one's own heart and mind, an internal sanctuary where one permits, respects, and cares for all they are. One must be connected with one's own deepest and most personal feelings, wishes, anxieties, shortcomings, and desires. If one does not know as much as one can about oneself, one has no anchor from which to evaluate, consider, and respond to all they see, all they hear, all that is peddled in their direction. They can only act as a sponge. As the ability to find oneself is not necessarily fueled by the intellect, there are plenty of brilliant sponges out there, perfectly disconnected from themselves, happily soaking it all in.

Unfortunately, when one's introspection muscle is never used, the very source of one's independent thought is made to atrophy. Only self-reflection fosters the self-possession that is required to think about things in whatever way one sees fit. In knowing oneself deficiently, what happens? The only thing that can: people begin to think in ways that others see fit, and they do so unknowingly. People begin to mistake independent thought for thought that is fully beholden.

For example, is a so-called original idea for an "app" an instance of independent thinking? After all, it is an idea for an app, which is perfectly unique to our values and context. A never-seen-before app that, I don't know, regrows hair, could be considered a product of independent thought in that novel ideas and calculations brought it into being. However, all of that novel thought was *determined* by prevailing notions of what makes thought valuable, which is to say, what makes it marketable (in this case, thought that yields the stimulation of hair follicles). Can determined and obedient thought be independent thought? Maybe, maybe not—you be the judge.

Relatedly, people interested in sociopolitical matters often take themselves to be independent thinkers because they have arrived at their own answers. But few consider that they have never arrived at their own questions, which are determined by massive institutions, prevailing values, and hundreds of other forces that determine exactly what tiny fraction of the world's goings-on will be deemed vital, important, and representative, to then be disseminated as "the" news. Despite what the average news consumer claims as independently derived opinions, as it relates to current events and cultural realities, he or she can only care about that which has *already been determined* to be worthy of their care; he or she can only think about that which has *already been determined* to be worthy of their thought.

Crucially, none of us has any measurable part in making determinations like these; what *does* have a part is our collective, unseen givens, which float around society, silently but faithfully hierarchizing its goings-on by relative importance, and yielding narratives about reality that are marketed, finally, as reality itself. This is not a "for or against" statement regarding any of the information available in society; rather, it is a *for reality* statement. It is too infrequently recognized that all of the varied narratives we could ever encounter on our screens, every last one of which *someone* would proclaim as reality, are less real than all the invisible processes, and all the values fueling them, by which they made their way to our screens (where, contrary to every prevailing view, actual reality has never and will never be found). Simply put, the information available to us is somehow not as real as whatever processes have made it—as opposed to something else—available to us.

Consequently, to have a thought about current events, whether it feels independent or not—and no matter its content—is to have been permitted that thought by every societal factor that helps determine what your consciousness will and will not be marinated in, from week to week. In fact, to the extent that all thought is embedded in some kind of culture and context, truly independent thought might be a fallacious concept, altogether. But if it were a true phenomenon, it might question its context relentlessly, or it might stand outside of it entirely, with little use for either its criticism or praise. Whatever the possibility of purely independent thought, however, one thing can be said about the most independent thinkers: they question themselves and, particularly, their own thought. What if we could look at the content of *our own minds* and see the question, or many questions, and not the answer? Unnatural as it sounds, then we'd *really* be thinking.

Compliance Culture

Unfortunately, as things stand now, because we aren't reflecting, we certainly aren't thinking independently; we're primarily "liking" and "disliking," reflexively. For this, there will be downstream effects. For example, on this trajectory, children will increasingly derive their ethics, their sense of what constitutes a just world, not from their own minds but from those making the best sale. The leveraging of undue social power is itself a new institution replacing reflective thought. While social influence has always existed, today's version is earned through means that are not only lacking in merit; they are often explicitly anti-merit. In 2022 we have finally just thrown our hands up and agreed that fame is cause for merit (when any capacity for reflection reveals that only the reverse could be true). Today, celebrity is the thing to be celebrated, and what's most important is being the most important. We should be able to say these things clearly, loudly, and freely because when we do, they can be addressed. And we should also be able to say we are much worse for all of this, maybe especially our youth.

It is becoming decreasingly true that kids learn from their teachers, their education, or even their families, all of which are institutions that, when working well, foster the ability to think for oneself. Increasingly, developing minds spend nearly all their time and garner nearly all their thoughts from the internet, a strange kingdom whose high rulers are those with the best websites, the most fans, and the raspberry tarts worthiest of parades. Thus, young people are more than just *susceptible* to encountering the self-promoted, self-marketed ideas of others—they are guaranteed to. The only world they've ever known is one made of information distributors, every one of whom specializes in distributing themselves, often with as much falsity as fervor.

As so much information flows so slickly and seamlessly, all of it cannot be thought about. Deliberate thought cannot catch up with all of it. Thus, as a strategy to gain the acceptance of peers, adolescents are better served by liking all the right things than by thinking through all the information available in order to learn what they *actually* like. In such a situation, social competency is somehow *genuinely* achieved via compliance. While history's adolescents also dealt with fitting in versus standing out, this tension is heightened for today's youth because so much of their lives are lived on social media, which is nothing but an ingroup-outgroup debacle of a very particular kind: the 24-hours-of-every-day kind. Kids can be rejected by peers at all hours of the day and night—and they know it. Consequently, the internal sanctuary I was mentioning above turns out to be especially unappealing to modern youth. Knowing how one *really* feels, what one *really* thinks, is a road, socially speaking, to nowhere, for healthy autonomy and self-possession could only get in the way of going along with the crowd. Even kids with naturally sturdy characters experience some version of this. They're kids, after all.

Good parents interested in promoting moral independence used to ask their adolescent, after he or she did some ill-advised thing with their peers, "Would you jump off a bridge just because your friend did?" In today's culture, posing this question turns out to be pretty risky, for it no longer has an obviously right answer. To today's child, it might well read as a test of their loyalty to the mob: "Yes, Mom and Dad. I'll do *anything* that has been deemed right by the possessors of good ideas! Is there a particular bridge I should like more than another?" Of course, this is not actually a joke. For everyone, the development of an internal moral compass is, with no exaggeration, of unparalleled seriousness.

So, what are the upper limits in a situation like this? To how much can one agree if they have almost no practice in generating their own attitudes and viewpoints? The answer should terrify all of us. If a person mistakes deference for the real use of cognition, there is simply no upper limit—none. If a "premier social influencer" wanted to, he or she has all the power to convince a substantial percentage of the US population, adults included, to start wearing one shoe to work, every Tuesday, starting next week. Reflexive compliance, otherwise known as unwitting obedience, is a first cousin of deficient introspection—and it knows no bounds. If you disagree, open any history book.

It is certainly troubling to acknowledge that the views children now claim as *their own* are often the views of their "favorite social influencer," a highly sought-after position in the modern world that, decoded, most often means "one with meritless power." But this is what happens to a developing mind when so many different ideas are pushed in its direction, complete with their own logos, websites, and marketing teams. Because the most common product in today's marketplace is this or that person's "brand," which, decoded, is just this or that person's view of the world, worldviews are now advertised like sneakers used to be. When I was 12, I wanted Air Jordan basketball sneakers because they were the best ones. I probably even hoped they would help me jump higher. Being sold a shoe, however, is quite a different thing than being sold a philosophy of life by a blogger with great hair and greater ambition.

In the first moment one steps foot on a basketball court, they learn that *suddenly acquiring* a new shoe is no substitute for skill. By contrast, one who *suddenly acquires* a new ideology from this or that "influencer" or "media personality" or "brand ambassador" will not so readily learn that adopting someone else's views is no substitute for genuine critical thought and contemplation. Unlike new sneakers, new worldviews are not tested in some tangible, behavioral world, akin to a basketball court. They are tested and retested on the internet, where they are guaranteed to find admirers, which means nothing of their soundness. In fact, as a mechanism for validating one's own thoughts, "the thoughts of others" has an illusion hiding in its very premise. What one thinks, including one who thinks they agree with me or you, *might* be a product of thinking; but it *might* just be a product of compliance or instinct or conviction or rage. To make matters worse, when one's views are made from any of the latter, they are often the last to know, thereby ruling themselves out as a serious source of feedback.

In fact, a person compromised in their ability to think critically, whatever the cause, is almost always obstructed from knowing it, since, by definition, they lack the very machinery that would permit them to evaluate the nature, depth, and intricacy of their own thinking. For this reason, a sense of blissful satisfaction with one's own thoughts is common in those missing the very equipment to further scrutinize them. This missing "equipment" is sometimes cognitive; that is, there are people who cannot think critically because they are not great at thinking. This is a simple reality of diverse intellects. But it isn't only limitations of cognition that obstruct people from thinking with more skill, scrutiny, and sophistication.

We have no idea how much anyone might improve at thinking, were they to develop a stronger relationship with themselves. In *really* appreciating the depths of something like the self, one becomes more schooled in the meaning of nuance, paradox, contradiction, and unavoidable complexity. In contacting oneself more fully and honestly, one finds a training ground for contending with complication, chaos, a lack of easy answers—and sometimes a lack of answers altogether. In successfully grappling with these properties of internal life, one somehow becomes more able to identify, appreciate, and think through the intricacies of many other problems. My view is that improved relations between self and self is our best hope not only for catalyzing higher quality thought but for overcoming every human problem that can be overcome, including 2022's gravest: the problem of being completely thoughtless with one another.

In Defense of the Humane

Being human is being complex, conflicted, convicted, fickle, high-minded, animalistic, and much more. We are all of it, and all of it informs all we do. We are so complicated that there is a vanity in even trying to explain the *why* behind what people say, think, feel, and do, for even if we have spoken continuously for an entire lifetime, we have not fully laid out all that drives someone. We might feel confident as to why Allie ended things with Patrick, or why our cousin likes a certain area of the country, or why our boss said that hostile thing; but what are these explanations when people are driven by so much we can't even see, let alone name? When it comes to people, being multidetermined means being an unknown quantity. Even hardcore social scientists would say so if you asked them about "effect sizes," which reveal that we understand next to nothing of what's inside the human motivation engine. Yet in everyday life, we can say why any given thing happened (just ask us). Short-circuiting this instinct is the beginning of reintroducing all that is humane. We simplify self and other, which is terminally detrimental to the humanity of both.

As we go through the world reducing other people and their motivations to *our explanations* of things, those explanations that are systematically most accessible *to us*, we are doing a grand disservice. We are forgetting that there is much more mystery to people, including ourselves; and in doing so, we are forgetting to be decent. This is why reflection is so dire: without delving deep into our own complexity, in all its divinity and darkness—and to be sure, there are wells upon wells of both—we forget to be good to each other. No human being really knows *exactly* what the hell they are doing; and they definitely don't know what others are. It's probably wiser to fear anyone who boasts otherwise than to "follow" them.

As we lose touch with the complexity of what it means to be human, inhumanity must emerge, sometimes in ways that seem unremarkable to us—but this only means we have become calloused. One version of such cruelty is a commonly acted out charade, the premise of which is that *we know*: we know what other people are, we know why they are what they are, and most dangerous of all, we know *what they should be*. When a person goes around treating other persons like they are supposed to *be a certain way, say a certain thing*, or *think a certain thought*, they have forgotten what people are—not least of whom, themselves.

Do other people come with guarantees to work in the very specific ways that suit us? Or have we, collectively and disastrously, confused our new neighbor with our new Jeep? There is probably no harm in expecting our $50,000 car to start each time we turn the key (probably), but we can't expect our neighbor, or ourselves, to be perfect and never corrupted; flawless and never fallible; patient and never surly; generous and never selfish; or diplomatic and never offensive. If we don't find improved ways of dealing with each other as we are, as we *really* are, society will surely self-destruct.

There might be nothing more deleterious to a society than citizens alienated from both themselves and others, yet we find ourselves trapped in a system that is not only speeding righteously at this outcome but proudly stepping on the gas, convinced to the bone that something good awaits. If any situation demands our sympathies, it's this one. Contemporary life is not a situation in which we human beings are passively losing our humanity; it's one in which we are being trained to throw it overboard. The only thing that can result is exactly what has: a total loss of respect for ourselves and each other. In a world where people's value for one another rests on factors it never should—the kind of clothes they wear, the "quality" of their last soundbite, the symmetry of their face, the number of people "following" them—we misunderstand what it means to be a person. This aspect of life, human relationships, is something we should be more interested in protecting, not merely "on paper," by way of phony, bureaucratic institutions like HR departments. We should *really care* about how we treat each other because it *really matters*.

This book, however, will not trace the development of our problems with reflection, critical thought, and undue faith in our own minds. It won't even elaborate these problems much further. Instead, it takes them as given characteristics of the modern psyche and responds with a distinct alternative. Our ways of understanding each other, whether through silly memes, sensationalized news stories, or our own personal knee-jerk attributions, desperately need revision. While this book is one about minds, psychotherapy, love, and change, it is just as much an act of burning defiance against the caricatured, shallow, and tired ways in which modern life encourages us to think about each other. In my view, we need to slow down and put some thought to our thought; some doubt to our certitude; some humility to our righteousness; and give more consideration to what we human beings really are. I hope this text contributes to these ends. While it is a small contribution and has very little chance of slowing the rising tide of brutality, superficiality, and insensitivity that defines our manner of treating one another, I'm writing it anyway because perhaps it will shift the thinking of a handful of people. Plus, if society is stuck in an undertow that will eventually drown the humanity in everyone, nothing would make me happier than being on record as a dissident.

In fact, you might take this book as my formal dissent against the anti-human sea in which we are now required to swim. It is full of reflection, thought, proposals, and offers many questions along the way for the reader's contemplation. My sincerest hope is that it serves as a stark corrective to our very human—but very misguided—sense that our own minds, by virtue of existing, have a monopoly on the assessment of reality. They certainly do not. The faster we can learn this, the faster we can treat one another with more respect. However, while this lesson requires thought to be learned, thought is not its takeaway point—something beyond thought is. Despite both my tone thus far and my clear appreciation for critical thinking, the thoughts that constitute this book have a somewhat paradoxical mission.

This book does not aim to promote thought for the sake of it, but rather, so that thought itself can be thought about—and so something very different can be seen. Despite its first aim, encouraging thought, and despite relying entirely on thought to make its case, this book does not make thought into the highest human good. To the contrary, it has a habit of making it into a source of illusion—something we overvalue, which results in the obstruction and not the discovery of the deepest knowns. The thought that constitutes this book is meant to move the reader beyond thinking and toward something else.

Intention Two: Beyond Thinking, in Favor of Something Else

In modern life, we say the world is what we say it is. We say that our way of seeing the world, operationalizing the world, and explaining the world *is the world*. We say that mystery is for fools who have not yet accepted that, through science, all questions go extinct. We say that a phenomenon that cannot be gripped by way of empirical methods is no phenomenon at all—or, at the very least, it isn't important or relevant. Science, the modern world's prized method of knowing, is built on unshakable faith in human perception and observation. And it permeates everything. Our tritest "memes" to our most respected experts tell us, with no shame or doubt, that science alone can explain everything worth explaining.

The scientific method, which is marketed as a synonym for ethical, advertises the superiority of the human mind as a kind of first principle. In a society where this assumption is so revered, it has a way of finding its way "into the water" so-to-speak. How could anyone drinking it *not* come to exalt their individual mind as supreme? I mean that as a serious question. Whether arrived at by way of genuine reflection and critical thought or by way of a lifestyle blogger's latest ramblings (and enviable linens), how could anyone do anything other than trust the conclusions that turn up in their own head? We have all learned that minds are the very path to unending knowledge, and if we're lucky, to utopia itself.

When looked at from this angle, people really shouldn't be criticized for taking the contents of their minds as blessed and the contents of other minds as profane. They have been taught that mind is king; and for each person, this could only mean their own. In turn, questioning one's own mind becomes an act of plain treason. And so, the misguided omniscience exhibited by people in every corner of society should not be attributed to their conceit or haughtiness, even if they seem to be these things, and even if they are. These days, thinking that people, including oneself, could know everything there is to know is not a problem of inflated ego, not primarily. It is first a problem of excessive obedience (which happens to be symptomatic of a lurking authoritarianism). It's to toe the party line; and in the current milieu, it's a fate no person can overcome without cognition prone to independence and scrutinization at the very least—if not outright revolt (which might be something I can help you with).

An Introduction to The Intrinsic World of Being

There exists a plane of human life that mind cannot reach. Not only is it the deepest aspect of reality; it's also the one we as modern people are required to undervalue. Where cognition has been made ultimate authority, that which is *too hard to understand* is rebranded, for the benefit of fragile egos, as that which one is *too intelligent to care about*. One who believes that reality is constituted precisely by that which he or she can grasp, operationalize, and consciously know, renders themselves impotent to find anything deeper—or even different—than their own thoughts. What follows from that is exactly what has: at the level of the individual, a flippant and unearned trust in one's own mind (despite knowing so little about it); and at the level of society, a collective ethos that everything is knowable. Even those skeptical of such an idea are insidiously and passively made to believe it as society rushes towards "*the real facts of everything*," a category to which we claim special access, and certainly more access than every tribe of people before us.

As for the text that follows, very little of it is about the problems of contemporary life; and none of it is meant to tear things down. It is meant to add something—to breathe life into things we have lost but desperately need to find once more. It is meant to help us return to humanity by putting forward a particular model of human experience, or at least the basis for one, which privileges something I call *the intrinsic world of being*. It is by way of this world that we can regrow respect for each other, build back mutual appreciation where there is now only antipathy, and more plainly, treat each other how we should.

The first feature of the intrinsic world is that while it can be talked about, as I am talking about it here, *it* can never be said. It is the aspect of human consciousness that is permanently confined to subjectivity, never to exit first-person experience: it exists there, only. It is therefore more intrinsic to human life than any possible *cognitive depiction* of human life. Thus, whatever the labels we ascribe to this world, whatever the methods by which we operationalize this world, *this world itself* remains wholly defiant of verbal capture. If one is talking about it or thinking about it, one is necessarily in touch with a version, representation, or replica of it, as opposed to *it itself*. Even naming it "the intrinsic world of being" violates is first property—it's inarticulability.

Thus, its name is not substantively important, for speaking of it at all makes it into something it cannot be—a construct. It is forever inexpressible because it isn't the stuff of the verbal world. It's that which can only be lived, never represented. Some people, owing to unwarranted faith in their cognitive and verbal apparatus, can hardly believe that all of subjectivity cannot simply be described. Thus, here is a quick way to distinguish that which can be operationalized and made into a construct from that which cannot.

You can tell me about experience, and I can take it as real and true. For example, you could tell me about a baseball game you went to with your family. In response, I can trust that your portrayal of the event reflects the actual event in some valid and important way. But despite your ability to tell me *about experience*, you can never *tell me experience*.

There's just no way to do the latter in words, which means that however honest you are in your depiction of the game, or anything else, it necessarily leaves something out. The next question is, what exactly does it leave out? Anything important? The answer fully depends on what you mean by "important." The modern world has generally dispensed with this aspect of human life for its reluctance to "get with the program." Because it does not bow to the intellect and refuses to be defined by the elaborate methods and systems that we have created for defining things, it cannot be especially important—or even especially real—as judged by prevailing values.

But let's (happily) drop prevailing values for a moment. What if all of us were in perpetual contact with this plane of human life, the one that we allege means nothing—and what if we all knew it? Then, what would it mean to claim that it isn't important, that it isn't *central* in understanding reality? Its default status as "negligible" would start to make less and less sense, when from this angle, it might be considered the *realest* thing there is. In turn, we would have to reconsider our approach to it. After all, it doesn't make logical or ethical sense to pretend something doesn't exist when it clearly does, solely because it behaves in a manner inconvenient to us and offensive to our sensibilities—this would be a little bit like pretending your best friend doesn't exist because he skipped your birthday party. Yet, the fact of its omnipresence is only the second-most compelling reason we human beings should think twice before dismissing the intrinsic world as important to human life.

Of foremost importance, the intrinsic world happens to be *all we share completely*; that is, it's the only thing we share in a way that is pure, perfect, and uncorrupted by mind because it does not permit access to mind, not directly. In fact, attempting to map this aspect of human life with thought, taxonomies, and systems requires us precisely to leave it behind. No such map *is* it; every such map *represents* it. This isn't to say that attempts to delineate the properties of human experience are ill-advised or that doing so only confuses us more. Sometimes taxonomy helps, and often it is necessary. For example, in psychotherapy, it is important to know whether your patient's consciousness is dominated by "rage" or "fear." Or in medicine, it is important to know if someone has asthma or a broken leg. There are plenty of classifications that we want to make, that we can make, and that help us. Classification systems are meant to guide us, and they can do just that. However, cognitively produced classification systems are undergirded by something we often fail to consider.

The Fleeting Nature of Mind-Derived Sameness

Bunching things together that go together does indicate sameness (e.g., Bill and Joe are both "X"). This sameness, however, owes itself to the existence of difference; in fact, all sameness does. This yields a strange implication for things our minds have classified as "the same," whether via elaborate methods of knowing or ordinary perception. So long as our minds have not lost any horsepower since grouping Bill and Joe as "X," their alleged sameness can never hold. Maybe they are the same on "variable X," but why would we think there aren't infinite subcategories of X, on which they differ? With mind as arbiter, sameness can never last: wheresoever there isn't today, tomorrow there will be difference.

This phenomenon is well represented in the natural course of scientific research, where classification is a never-ending enterprise. For example, no heart attack is just a heart attack; it's a subtype of a heart attack. What's more, heart attacks of the same category will eventually differ, even if we do not yet know how. We know this because existing research that digs further into currently understood mechanisms and processes aims, by definition, to *know more*, which means, *to make further distinctions*. The 30,000-foot-view looks like this: if we could know everything about every person's body—and we soon might—there would be no general "disease process" that yields "heart attacks." Instead, there would be as many disease processes as individuals—no more and no less. If we knew enough, we might even be able to assign a weight to every moment of every person's life, reflecting its relative contribution to their longevity versus decline. Every single second could be characterized.

Here is my point. When the mind's powers of observation, scrutiny, and discernment reach their peak, not only is no heart attack like any other heart attack; ultimately, *no thing* is like *any other thing*. Every item contained within the same category must eventually become a category unto itself. This is to say that classifications aren't final. This can be seen in day-to-day life, in the most mundane ways. Can you remember a day where, per your mind, Mexican food was "the best," only to be moved into the "lukewarm" category a few months later? Are there weeks wherein you see yourself as basically peaceful on Tuesday but short-tempered by Friday? Are there summers in which you view yourself as content, only to find yourself desperately hoping for more pleasure, more joy, more aliveness by November?

Whether a subcomponent of a disease process across cardiology patients, personality traits thought to be shared by new friends, or a view of oneself over time, all the "sameness" that the mind has derived, all the sameness defined by the mind's belief in it—*any mind-produced sameness*—is an illusion. It is not evidence that things are the same but evidence that further processes of mind have not yet been unleashed, for when they are, they will rip things apart. The mind, a rabid, drooling dog, will further differentiate, classify, and sort everything it touches. Sameness found by minds must be lost. From trite to profound, from food preferences to ethical ideals, that which a person *thinks* they share with others is sure to collapse—if not with this person, then with the next; that which a person *thinks* defines them is sure to collapse—if not today, then tomorrow. The mind, by its nature, is a vehicle for further and further discrimination. And it's supposed to be—no one on their way to the hospital with "some kind of heart issue" would have it any other way. The mind classifies, unendingly.

Toward Each Other

More than an attempt to foster thought, this book is an attempt to resituate the intrinsic world of being—all that cannot be operationalized—as primary, as the absolute bedrock of human life, because as I will explain, this reads to me as the only viable way toward the good. The modern worldview is not merely intellect-centered; it is intellect-reverent. For all its benefits, this arrangement is insidiously disconnecting. In modern life, including modern psychology, we are forgetting that there is more to life than cognition. While we have been programmed to take the intellect and all its discerning power as wholly good, it also happens to hold the most potential to wreak havoc on human life. Today, the mind has convinced itself that, *by way of itself*, it can alter human beings, constitutionally and for the better. Yet, despite society's vainglorious goal of engineering human perfection, and despite the obedience and conformity that fuels its proponents, human beings cannot be perfect, nor can they be made to be the same, not in the most manifest realm, anyway; what's more, in the *realest* realm, we already are, always have been, and always will be the same. Unfortunately, one who believes we ought to be the same on every observable characteristic is in for what might seem to them like the rudest of awakenings, but it's only an awakening to reality.

Human beings are different. As such, we will offend each other. We will harm each other. We will destroy things that should only ever be protected. We will fight like animals, and still learn nothing from each other. We will wish we had changed sooner. We will wish the best of people could be perfect, which they can't. We will act our frustration and hatred over things that are actually good enough, well-intentioned, or even just right. We will think we are more talented than we are. We will think others are less talented than they are. We will be envious, murderous, and shortsighted—and especially when we feel most right-eous, most unreceptive to caution or prudence. We will commit to never doing certain things again; then, we will do them again—and again; then we will convince ourselves that we didn't *really* want to stop doing them anyway. What do we do about this? All I claim to know, when it comes to our shared and natural corruption, is what we must not do, not under any circumstance: we must not fancy ourselves executioners. We must not kill each other off in our hearts and minds for the fact of our imperfections, our *shared* imperfections. If we did that, there would soon be no one left, as being human is being imperfect. What humans are meant to do and must do is to *coexist despite*—despite different values, different histories, different cultures, different intellects, and all the other differences that can only be missed by egregious and willful blindness.

Unfortunately, our shared reverence for mind, a tool whose function is discrimination, has made coexistence harder and harder to achieve these days. In the moment science, rationality, or any other systematic method of knowing gets off the ground, difference emerges in the expression of variables and constructs— forms that are distinct from other forms. Our minds set out to know what the world is and what it isn't; who is X and who is Y; and which notions hold water, and which don't. Right now, why are you reading this text, and not pouring your coffee into it? Because the mind, a tool that naturally splinters the world into X and Y, has deemed it a book, not a coffee mug.

Not only is hyper-classification fundamentally *right* per our troubled values; it's also fundamentally *unavoidable* regardless of them. After all, in everyday life, none of us could do without our judgements any more than an ER doc could upon encountering a cardiac patient. But distinction-making has become a cognitive reflex, an uncontrolled spasm that prevents us from being still enough to see the possibility of something more foundational, a unity made not from the latest-breaking set of facts, nor any other products of mind to which we have agreed (for the time being). No, robust unity will not be found across minds, which are the most sophisticated tools for division that the world will ever know; nor will it be found across that which minds create, since all things borne of mind— including ideas, opinions, preferences, and values—can vary across people. The terrain of mind, after all, is a terrain of difference.

Thus, a world that expects unity but reveres the intellect either doesn't really expect unity or doesn't understand cognition, which is not a tool for unity. One might think, "wait, but I can use my mind to think my way to the value of unity." Good for you—and other people can use theirs think their way to something totally different. For this reason, holding some expectation that the content of our fellow man's mind *ought* to look like the content of ours is not just perfectly inhumane; it reveals an exquisitely dangerous misunderstanding. Anything one mind can see, another mind can see differently. One who refuses this, or pretends it isn't so, or feels strongly that it should be different, is always within spitting distance of misanthropy. Minds, before they do anything else, vary.

It is Not Our Minds that Binds Us

Some time ago I became oddly attuned to the possibility that difference itself might be a terribly destructive illusion, despite that people, our minds, and the world are all seemingly defined by it. Ultimately, it is an illusion. But learning so involves learning that the mind is an incompetent teacher. This is very hard to grip, especially for people with well-working minds, perhaps most especially for prideful intellectuals who are unable to understand why everyone doesn't just think like they do. Nonetheless, in order to understand each other as we really are—*the same*—we cannot look to the mind. Minds are different and they are meant to be. They will not teach us of sameness. They will not teach us that everything billowing around the internal landscape of the other is so too billowing around ours. Nor will they teach us of the other's humanity, not fully or always, because other people are something more than mind can grip—and so are we.

Just don't look to your mind for confirmation. For every genuine achievement that belongs to it, ranging from modern sanitation to electricity to the internet, the thinking, analyzing, discriminating mind has always been and always will be an unmitigated failure in its capacity to teach us about something deeper than itself. It thinks it can teach us about the world, but it can never see the things it cannot see. Not only that—it can never see that there *are things* it cannot see. Yet, its foremost assumption, the one undergirding all its output, is that it has seen everything, that it has taken account of everything seeable. This feature of mind makes it the *sine que non* of human arrogance.

Anything to which the mind applies itself, no matter how homogenous *seeming*, will soon be delineated and diced up into parts, thus kickstarting distinction and introducing heterogeneity. However, in the matter of consciousness *itself*, in the matter of first-person experience *itself*, taxonomization does not make difference; it appears to, but it cannot do so because its tool—verbal depiction—cannot reach deep enough into subjectivity to fracture it. Imagine that, per our taxonomies, I am "high functioning," and you are "severely anxious." In the world of representation this makes us different. However, when we represent subjectivity with language, segment it, then allocate some of its parts to you (severely anxious) and others to me (high functioning), that which binds us has still not been broken—because that which binds us was never amenable to verbal segmentation nor representation *in the first place*.

Even if the properties of mine would be described differently than the properties of yours per our taxonomies, and even if mine and yours contained different qualities, consciousness *is* as much for me as it *is* for you. And here's the kicker: if we want to be *really* honest, that's all that can be said about *it*, since the first moment in which we carve up and represent subjectivity, activities which instantiate apparent division between me and you, is the very moment in which the thing we are after disappears before our eyes. In describing the subjective experience of consciousness, one turns it into something other than itself—a mere likeness of it, which is not *it*. Thus, before investigations by thought into subjective experience show us what it is, they adulterate it, thereby abandoning it.

In this sense, taxonomizing and classifying hinge on a usually unseen paradox. Without question, these processes hold tremendous power to create discrete buckets. Take psychiatry, for example, wherein "anhedonia" goes in the "depression" bucket. These buckets, because they help us know an enormous amount *about* people, are assumed to help us better understand them, to help us better grasp or reach them. But if the reader has followed me, he or she can probably guess what's on the other side of the paradox: how exactly could imposing difference, where there was not difference previously, foster *more* understanding? As far as the conceptualizing mind is concerned, yes, processes of taxonomizing and classifying mean more knowing; in another way, though, they mean disconnecting people from one another. These processes find the very substance by which people were connected without trying to be, the stuff of consciousness itself, and they intervene into it—with a sledgehammer. While such processes are helpful for conceptual knowing (e.g., "person A is depressed, not paranoid"), they also sever *precisely* that which tethers people to each other.

First-person experience, and particularly the aspect of it which cannot be operationalized—the intrinsic world—is unbreakably shared. This makes it unique, for every other thing that holds potential to be shared will be shattered when thought and language—*when mind*—enter the scene. But so is not the case with that which is permanently intrinsic to *being itself* because it is a realm into which mind cannot find its way. It is a realm permanently confined to subjectivity itself, never to be verbally or cognitively captured. Unlike the world of mind, where differences grow like weeds, the intrinsic world of being is a plane in which difference evaporates. But even more than that, it's a place where difference never was, as it is a place where mind has never been. Thus, it maintains a special, even sacred function. When we have lost each other, it must be the only way back to one another. The intrinsic world must be the only rightful bridge.

Thinking Through (a Representation of) The Intrinsic World

Now, what does it mean that people share something that cannot be captured with words or thoughts? For one, it might mean that asking such a question is self-contradictory: how could the mind answer questions about a domain defined by its absence? Maybe it can't; maybe the mind is not the vehicle for answering such questions. My sense is that it isn't. But for many, the mind's inability to answer a question rules out that very question as a question at all, or at least as a worthwhile one; from such a perspective, that which cannot be answered with mind was never a question to begin with. And this view is fair enough. After all, if you're keeping up *at all* in the modern world, you know that a phenomenon the intellect cannot grasp is no phenomenon at all (or alternatively, it's one we just haven't captured yet).

Here is another, difficult question: if there really is a domain of experience that we cannot represent in thought and language, even if we can talk *about it* or think *about it*, what impact might it have on all the things we *can* legitimately say or think. At bottom, this question asks: how does something we can only experience and never "think up" contribute to all we do "think up?" Of course, this question suffers from the same problem alluded to above, since it presupposes the mind as the answerer, when, in fact, it would be a conundrum with which the mind has no first-hand experience so-to-speak. All the mind really knows of the intrinsic world is an after-the-fact, thought-generated analogue, since "the intrinsic world proper" is unreachable with mind. What our minds know of the moments and processes that have constituted being is something distinct from being itself. The primary characteristic of the intrinsic world is that mind is nowhere to be found therein.

Nonetheless, despite being inaccessible with thought, this domain of life somehow has access to us, always, in every passing moment, as it is intrinsic to experience and life itself. This begins to turn the tables a bit with respect to the usual sense of power we grant our minds. Think and think as we might, we won't find the intrinsic; yet somehow, it is always there. This is a kind of first clue for contacting it, whatever it is. In order to better grip this deepest aspect of human experience, we must somehow delve further not into cognition but into something else, something that is not thought and cannot be thought.

This process could be reasonably called different things, though the word "inwardness" has always made the most sense to me, as this pursuit is firstly a pursuit of one's own inward ground. But it only starts out that way. What it leads to is something bigger, better, and so profound as to eclipse any data about the self. Eventually, from going within oneself, other things emerge, things that are explicitly non-self in nature—less personal and more transpersonal. Over time, a commitment to inwardness reveals what *being is*, rather than what *one is*; and strangest of all, it isn't one's mind but one's being that learns.

This Book's Central Proposition

Confessions and Disclaimers

As laid out in the *Preface*, my interest in human experience was not initially academic nor intellectual. It was very personal. Nonetheless, once these interests had gripped me, I sought out more learning—first on my own in New York area libraries, and then more formally in academic psychology. While I have never taken a philosophy class, I have dabbled in a certain brand of thinker; namely, the kind who delights in taking nothing as given. First it was Schopenhauer for his insistence that the world registers as a matter of something that is part and parcel of life itself, then the Eastern traditions for related reasons. These perspectives compounded my already deep interest in subjective experience and moved me to clinicians like Heinz Kohut and Carl Rogers, the latter of whom constructed a paradigm so elegant in its simplicity that the bottomlessness of its depth is often lost on people. I have also found my way into the thought of existentialists, most importantly, Kierkegaard, who appears to have handily mapped the stages of my life long before it started.

The truth, though, is that in arriving at what I think, I never looked too deeply into anyone else's thoughts. I was just never looking for anyone else's thoughts; I was only ever looking for my own, and I always knew it. This might well be a character flaw, but especially considering where I landed, it also aligns me more squarely with one tradition than all others, one that is varied, hetero-geneous, and consequently not perfectly coherent as a category. My outlook sees something beyond mind, and therefore might aptly be termed "mystical."

Yet, you are not about to read a book of ghost stories. I take myself to be as committed to reality as a person can be. In fact, it's *because of* this very trait that I don't blindly take reality as something human beings can just readily and easily grip—this obviously incudes myself. In fact, it has always seemed to me that the most *realistically* based view of reality would have to be the one that makes the most room for that which might well lie beyond it. In other words, when the unspeakable complexity of the world is seen rightly, it becomes clear that without being committed to humility, one cannot be committed to reality. There's too much we don't know; too much we can't know; too much we might never know.

The mystical tradition stands not just for the importance of raw experience; it knights raw experience and internal life as the very path to truth. Despite growing from different religions and eras, mystics have quietly offered the same message throughout human history: in order to find the deepest realities in the world, we must go looking in the deepest parts of ourselves. All of this is offered as a confession to the reader. Despite all my education, formal and informal, all my clinical interactions, and all my conversations with people in and around my field, some of whom embody a giftedness so given that it doesn't register until they've left the room, before this book is anything else, it is the product of simple inwardness. I say so here because it is truest of the book's central idea, which in its primordial form, was not an idea at all.

This book's major proposition is a suggestion as to how the unconceptualizable world, which is unreachable with mind, impacts the functioning of minds, nonetheless, including the manner in which minds conceptualize and formulate. It is a suggestion as to how cognition (i.e., how we attend to, perceive, and interpret), including all we can say, think, and explain about these processes, is subordinate to something we can never say or think, subordinate to some aspect of experience that might be said to exist permanently "behind the mind's back" so-to-speak, as it can never be captured with cognition. In other words, this book's major proposal is that something the mind cannot conceptualize governs all its conceptualizing apparatus. In attempting to bridge the unconceptualizable aspect of human experience with human conceptualization, it poses a way in which the human mind, and all it thinks, is impacted by something it *cannot think*. Now the reader can probably see the elephant standing in the middle of this book's central idea.

The truth is that I cannot describe what I'm trying to because anything I say is forever a product of the very process whose origins I'm trying to map. The way in which one's conceptualizations of the world are brought forth is an *activity* to be experienced, apprehended, or felt from within the confines of one's own subjective experience before it is a set of ideas or a model to be represented. This is necessarily the case if one understands that thinking about "how one conceptualizes" is showing up late to the party (since one already has). That which moves one to conceptualize vanishes in the very same moment one thinks about that which moves one to conceptualize; in its place, always, are the fruits of conceptualization, never the seeds.

Because this is a book, however, and because I hope to convey something to other minds, the bridge that links the unconceptualizable world with the conscious conceptualizations we hold in mind must be offered in the form of language. That is, in the service of communication, a process that never exists in cognition will be verbally elaborated in the text that follows, which means a couple of equally strange things about reading this book. First, even if the link between unconceptualizable and conceptualizable, as offered in the text, makes *cognitive sense* to the reader, this is still no criterion for its validity or its existence. The process *as it takes place* does not exist in thought, even if the process as represented in thought comports with the reader's sense of rationality and reason (which I hope it does). For this process, its true validity criterion exists in the domain of that which is exclusively experienced, not represented in mind. It exists internal to each reader. The second and related oddity of this situation is that the author sets out to show something to the reader, knowing full-well that even the best "proof" cannot touch the process meant to be proven, for it exists outside the scope of proof as we normally mean it.

This is all said so that reader and writer can, together, acknowledge and resolve an unavoidable shortcoming within the central proposition of this book. It will knowingly put concepts to the unconceptualizable as a matter of necessity. However, this also points at the best way to utilize the book. There is something more to do, beyond cognitively comprehending all that is put forth. There is also something to be apprehended—an experiential analogue to find within oneself. And so, no point in this book is meant to be "final." Stranger still, no point in this book can prove what it aims to. The best it can do is point the reader in the direction of something that will only be found, internally. Simply enough, as much as I can lay out the "mechanics" of the intrinsic world, and as much as they might "make sense" to those reading, they can only ever actually be experienced.

This text offers a sense as to *how minds* are *made*—how people come to see, think about, and conceive of the world; and of special importance, the role that an unseeable, unthinkable, inconceivable domain of human experience has in *making them*. At the base of this book is the author's thoroughgoing and unyielding sense that something extremely consequential goes on in a world we cannot think—and that it goes on for all of us. I call it a "sense" only because calling it an intuition makes it sound that much flimsier (and I want the reader to continue trusting me, assuming they've not already stopped). Now, I'd like to lay out the process that defines the intrinsic world; while it takes the form of an idea to be understood below, in its most native form, it is an internal activity to be found.

"The Investing Process"

We might say that the intrinsic world of being is a world of investment, as it houses an ongoing *investing process* that takes place beyond conscious mind.

By way of this process, we make investments in what subjective experience will be—in what being will be, in what consciousness will be. We are not privy to our investments, however, because remember, all of this takes place in a domain inaccessible to thought, which is to say, we do not use our minds to conclude how subjective experience ought to be, then somehow make it that way. This reads true when we reflect on what it's like to be alive. Nobody feels that the quality of their own, first-person experience was something in which they had a hand; it feels much more like it simply formulated itself, like it was just there to be embraced (or bothered by). While the conditions of subjectivity are different for different people (e.g., some people are often sad while others are often content), the process by which it develops—i.e., the process by which subjectivity becomes what it eventually becomes—does not vary across people.

I do not mean this in the way a strict empiricist would: that a particular set of variables (those related to genes, culture, and interpersonal history) come together to create each of our idiosyncratic, psychological outcomes. Empirically, this is true. Certain variables are in fact so weighty that they help account for the course of every human life. But the actual terrain of human experience, and especially its most *intrinsic* domain, as it defies conceptualization, contains no variables. It contains no facts. From this perspective, the empirical formula that claims to explain the development of subjectivity and personhood, the one that includes facts about biology, environment, and so on, necessarily counts out everything that might contribute to one's quality of subjectivity *from within subjectivity*. It counts out all that is native and confined to subjectivity, all that refuses to be "factualized" or "propositionalized" or "conceptualized" that might, nonetheless, contribute to subjectivity as it now stands. In order to count this material back in, there is simply no tool like that of the self, no aid like that of going inward. This is how all of us find the investing process as it operates internal to us.

The Fruits of Inwardness: Encountering the Investing Process

When one first goes into the being world, a non-language world, one finds what might be called "the sense of suffering," and one finds it with an almost offensive ease. Yet, enough time spent with the nature of being reveals that despite its unavoidability, the being world is not *made of* suffering, for even suffering grows from something more fundamental than *it*. When one goes far enough inward, when one burrows deep enough into the world unreachable with thought, something is encountered that is so loud as to deaden every other sound, so bright as to render colorless every competing sight, and so sharp as to pierce and infiltrate one's every cell. Something is encountered that is *so true* as to falsify, in some fundamental and undeniable sense, every other thing. In the deepest inwardness, one finds the nethermost substance of which the being world is made. The world we cannot contact with our minds, but occupy even so, is made of something that despite having no good verbal corollary, can only be appropriately called, *love*. If that claim feels spurious at best—and more than that, close to unhinged—it's because I'm putting language to something for which there are no good words. And yet, there's more.

With inwardness, one finds that love is not merely a quality that swirls around and exists *in* the being world; rather, one finds that its relative presence versus absence *defines* the being world, *constitutes* the being world, *is* the being world. Thus, it is always there in some capacity, even if only in the form of relative absence; therefore, it is always leaving its mark on people—*differentially so*. Although our minds cannot scan this world, for they cannot enter it, some other aspect of us, forever confined to our being, can and does. Then, it responds.

This is where the investing process, briefly introduced above, the one to which we are not cognitively privy, is set in motion. The relative nature of one's contact with love, including not only its availability versus scarcity but also the form in which it is brought to bear, causes one to invest in *being certain things* and *not others*; it causes one to invest in a manner of being marked by *these* tones, flavors, and textures, not *those* ones. Simply enough, the nature of one's relative contact with love causes one to invest in a consciousness marked by *this*, not *that*; and of special importance, this investment takes place with *no assistance from thought*. Therefore, we cannot be cognitively aware of this investing process as it happens, nor can we track it with cognition, once it has.

However, there is one aspect of this process of which we are distinctly and continually aware: its consequences, which manifest *in and as* conscious mind. It is from our investments, those we have made in what subjectivity will be, that our whole manner of conceptualizing—the idiosyncratic manner by which we come to take as true that which we take as true—is born. This means that even if our minds are different, which they certainly are, they have been made different by a process that we share, permanently. The investing process is what anchors us to each other, even if in running its course, it yields exquisitely different minds. This is to say that what bonds us, eternally and without exception, is the manner in which the very substrate of reality has touched us. Sure, love has made our minds *different*, but it has made them, *nonetheless*.

All of this has implications not only for how we might understand the mind of the other but for how we might best *treat* the other. The content of our minds, of which we are so sure and trust so faithfully, implicitly, and unreservedly, owes itself to something else, a process of investment that operates precisely where mind isn't. And so, whether we want to *understand other people,* which we do if we want to be humane, or *alter other people's knowns,* which we do if we are therapists (recall the *Preface*), we must see the mind as something like a dead end, a temptation that can get us only so far. The willfully accessed mind as we know it is not the seat of consciousness; and therefore, it will not be the seat of change. The mind is a ripple on the surface, and we all know it, don't we? The mind is not·at the bottom of life, and we all know it, don't we?

Implications

And so, the major purposes of this book are two. The first is simple. I want the reader to think and reflect. This is radical enough, given current times and modern minds. Yet the book's other purpose is to encourage a kind of thought that is perhaps less acceptable still, at least as the modern world is concerned. As a matter of complete and total transparency, this text's second and more ambitious purpose is less a pursuit for the good of clinical psychology and related fields, and much more a pursuit for the good of the author's own heart.

I want to relocate the most important aspect of human life—important to understanding self and other, and to treating each other humanely. Although we can never put words to it, the deepest and truest world in which all of us live and with which all of us are in eternal contact is not the world of our own cognition but the intrinsic world of being. These worlds are different but related: the goings-on of the former, which cannot be conceptualized, account for the goings-on of the latter, which consist of conceptualization. For this, there are major upshots, most of which clinical psychology cannot see, since most of clinical psychology, co-opted by scientism, cannot see how anything that truly exists could possibly defy conceptualization. Consequently, where there might otherwise be something substantive and real, our field continues to find only cheap tricks and gimmicks, which we are satisfied can intervene into the deepest, most important parts of people. Unfortunately, this is a misunderstanding that puts in peril both the field and the human beings for whom it cares.

People are not helped by the "accurate delivery of valid interventions" because people are not machines. People do not become more effective when administered the "newest, state-of-the-art technologies" because people are not computers. People do not change by having their thought "restructured" because people are not merely minds. What people *are*, most fundamentally, is something that refuses to be uttered, but the descriptor—*soul*—has always seemed sufficient to me. And the world that souls inhabit—the intrinsic world—as it is ruled by only one quality, knows only one currency.

In these terms, what it might mean for any one person to help any other person, whether a therapist and patient, parent and child, or two strangers in a chance encounter, shows itself with a spellbinding clarity. Whatever else it means, whatever else *we say* it means, it must also mean—it must first mean—*the unqualified addition of love*. I have my way and you have yours; but as far as I can see, this must be the purpose of psychotherapy and life itself.

PART I

The Basis for a Critique

1

BEYOND THE WORLD OF CONSTRUCTS

This book is written for the fields of psychiatry, psychology, social work, and all others whose purview is human distress; however, it could probably be utilized by anyone curious about minds in relationship, which is the very basis of not only the helping professions but life itself. I am writing this book because in the very same fields whose work is defined by it, the mind is becoming decreasingly appreciated. At first blush, this trend might not be so obvious; after all, the mind appears to be the focus of all our efforts. For example, we put our interventions to use only after having characterized someone's mind as "depressed" or "paranoid." We also measure and categorize relative anguish by the contents of a person's mind (e.g., we might identify "generalized anxiety" when the course of a person's thinking is much too fear-laden, much too often). In these ways, we do seem devoted to the mind. It seems to be the very seat of our work.

The trouble is that in thinking about it so often, with so little effort and so much reflex, we have made a caricature of the single most complicated facet of human life. We act as if the human mind was made for—and is even defined by—all the constructs we have introduced into its orbit (e.g., depression, cognitive therapy, bipolar disorder, anger management, and all the rest). In orienting to the mind in this way, it becomes just another stale construct, the defining feature of which is its amenability to "quick and easy understanding." Making the mind into a construct not only gives us a rote, scripted understanding of what it really is; doing so also gives us permission to stop thinking about what it really might be. This situation, in which our field now finds itself, has its causes, some more warranted than others and some of which a book could never resolve, but their cumulative effect is to create and reward thoughtlessness about what it is that we are doing. If people meant to deal with human problems are not being trained to

DOI: 10.4324/9781003305286-3

contemplate the meaning of the human mind, what are they being trained to do? Unfortunately, the answer is: something much more superficial.

The State of The Field

Implicit throughout the mental health field is a system of identifying human problems and assigning them importance as a matter of their relative perceptibility. Simply, we see problems as that which we can see. This might not appear so unreasonable at first glance. In fact, it takes no time at all to think of an example in which the most observable problem and the most pressing problem are one and the same. For example, if a patient is cutting themselves every night and discussing in therapy every method by which they might commit suicide, there are no problems more pressing than these—and they are the most evident. Relatedly, there is an associated version of clinical care that, when abided by with good intention, is nearly impossible to find fault with. Who could argue with this patient's clinician over their wholehearted and hell-bent commitment to fix these problems at nearly any cost? I have watched this very dynamic take shape in ways I have found altogether beautiful. We are concerned with the most observable problems because they often matter.

However, when that which is most observable most informs our understanding of the problem, the entire concept of "problem" changes before our very eyes. It becomes systematically restricted. What is readily observable and what is thought to be going wrong become so tied up together as to lose distinction; and in turn, factors that are less than visible—however relevant or related to the issue at hand—are missed. From there, several unseen consequences follow, which together result in a clinical bent defined by its lack of depth. We end up thinking in a stereotyped way about human problems and what it might mean to solve them.

In doing so, we arrive at the most simplistic of all possible views as to the relationship between the purpose of therapy and the problem at hand: the goal of treatment is nothing more than a reduction in the problem's frequency. That is, "presenting problem" and "treatment goal" are the same phenomenon, only happening at different rates, moving at different clips. Under this scheme, we already know what treatment should *do*, well before giving any thought to what it might *be*: it should change the incidence of this or that problem. All of this might sound perfectly reasonable; however, the difficulty sets in when we take the 30,000-foot perspective of things. From this altitude, there is something we cannot help but see, something we didn't see before.

Our psychotherapeutic treatments are not exactly reducing problems. They are reducing problems that we have defined as such and to which we have ascribed importance. They are reducing only the problems we have *observed as problems*. It is important to state here that my contention is not that treatment modalities following this formula are useless. For example, a patient who panics twice a day will certainly feel better if, after attending eight sessions of cognitive behavioral therapy (CBT), he or she find themselves panicking only twice per month. This is a great outcome. Life is better lived without acute anxiety, so aiming to diminish it makes perfect sense. I am only pointing out that our view of the "treatment process" from start to finish—from the disorder we identify, to the intervention we employ, to the way me measure improvement—has much to do with us. It would have to, given that we created it. Failure to acknowledge our hand in things is how we first forget the mind in favor of the constructs that stand in for it. Let me explain.

The general human pursuit to know the world and uncover its mechanisms is a process that rests on our capacity to observe. In psychology, we allege that the component of the world we are most interested in observing is experience. But the yield of any observational process aimed at capturing human experience is not equivalent to the experience itself; though rampantly overlooked, it tells us nothing about the quality of the experience and everything about its correlates. For example, we know that changes in appetite and sleep, decreased motivation, and low mood are correlated with what we call depression. Yet we could know every correlate of this state, including its brain-based, interpersonal, and affective manifestations, and still know nothing of the state itself. As features of human experience become sufficiently salient as to earn our interest, we create their language-derived analogues, thereby situating them in terms that make them understandable to us, and at the very last moment we do something we really shouldn't. We claim that rather than having created our constructs, we discovered them.

This results in the widely accepted notion that upon identifying all the existing characteristics and correlates of depression—everything derived at the limits of observation that is amenable to language—we know all there is to know about it. If you listen carefully, you can hear the empiricist cheer, "We have found what we are looking for!" But this is a misstep. Constructs are not discovered, not entirely. They are also constructed. Nonetheless, in a certain way, such a cheer is entirely defensible, for this brand of investigation into depression can teach us nearly everything about *what it is*. Unfortunately, it holds no such potential to teach us *what it's like*. This might sound strange to some readers who have never questioned the very basis of their field—the nature and utility of its favorite concepts—but I hope you hear me out.

Something like depression is firstly an experience, and only secondarily, its language-situated offshoots—its "correlates," "manifestations," and "criteria," for example. This is seen clearly in how it is researched, where the first matter of business must always be experience. For example, to identify characteristics of a depressed brain, it is essential to study the brains of people experiencing a certain thing. If they are not experiencing that thing, or appropriate levels of it, we conclude that they are not depressed and therefore hold little utility in helping us understand depression. Depression is a construct, like all psychological constructs, defined by particular characteristics of *being*. It would be backward to conclude the opposite—that it came into existence primarily by way of its correlates (e.g., changes in brain chemistry, interpersonal manifestations, cognitive changes), and only secondarily, by the experiential state. Not only does empirical investigation bear a different order in that meaningful correlates follow from specific states; so too does human life. To name an aspect of experience or to identify its correlates, one must first *encounter the thing, in being*. Experience precedes and gives rise to the identification of experience.

If this is taken to be true, psychological constructs owe their existence to subjectivity; by way of observation, the former is meant to capture the latter. However, this observational process has a strange way of leading our attention away from what initially drew it—experience—and toward something else. This is due in part to competing human processes. The process required to *grip* the quality of an experience is very different from the one required to elaborate it, verbally and cognitively. However, upon devoting our attention to anything, including human experience, we innately engage the latter process, thanks to our verbal nature. We can't help it; we identify, elaborate, and categorize, instinctually. So, we first become interested in a particular state of being, and we then go looking into it. What we find is an ungodly amount of information about the subjective state of interest. To demonstrate this point, just consider everything you know about depression. You can probably identify its cognitive, emotional, and interpersonal implications, its various courses, the role of genes in its development, and much more. While this is useful information, it does not represent a step toward the realm of the subjective, which is what prompted our interest in the first place. It can only represent a step to the side, into a nearby realm that might be called something like, "facts about the subjective."

This is the realm that teaches us about sleep disturbance, distortions in thinking, problems in motivation, and all the rest. If it seems hard to believe that this is not the stuff of subjectivity, even though it represents the verbal depiction of various subjective phenomena, ask yourself why you were not reluctant to call to mind every known characteristic of depression for fear that it might send you into a depressive spiral. The answer is obvious: saying or thinking about "anhedonia" is not a risk factor for losing interest in life. That it could be is obviously a ridiculous idea, but the reason it's so ridiculous should not be overlooked because it betrays a hard truth, unacknowledged through and through in psychology. Our constructs, which represent our best scheme to capture experience, are entirely bereft of experiential meaning. I am not claiming that things should be otherwise, but rather, that they never could be. First-person experience and the language through which we aim to capture it are made of different materials.

Imagine what would happen, though, if the clinical world regularly confused these things; that is, if upon identifying and categorizing experience, we fancied ourselves already operating in the realm of subjectivity, almost as if *facts about subjectivity* provided us access to *subjectivity itself*; or relatedly, if we conflated our *words for experience* with *experience itself*. This might mean that the act of psychotherapy, which is thought to apprehend, intervene into, and ultimately improve human experience, could operate with almost no regard for subjectivity, and not know it. We could identify the most observable clinical issue and conclude that because we have the apt descriptor, we also understand the problem. Next, an explosion of thought would take place in the "facts about subjectivity" realm, resulting in our total understanding of the problem's characteristics. Only a few short seconds later, we could identify both the treatment goals and the treatment plan best suited to the problem. We could do all of this—fully understand the problem, identify treatment goals, and plan an entire course of treatment in order to improve a patient's experience—with almost no investigation into the experience itself. For efficiency's sake, we could put out a single workbook to treat the depression of millions of different people and feel earnestly convinced that our scope of interest is individual experience—that is, *the subjectivity of individual persons*. We might even feel confused if someone dare claim otherwise. After all, we are in the field of psychology. We must care about the psyche, right? No; this is, of course, empty logic. The state of psychology cannot be ascertained by way of its label any more than the state of depression.

Some might argue, however, that current practices in psychology are warranted because the goal of treatment is not necessarily to delve into idiosyncratic experience but to alleviate symptoms. Even clinicians who consider themselves "non-medical model" sometimes see it this way—that our primary task is to make the symptoms go away and, in order to do so, circumscribed and targeted treatments can suffice. That we want symptoms as we know them to go away is not the question (of course, we do). The question is, "how do we know symptoms?" What exactly are symptoms? As symptom alleviation models gain traction, symptoms are increasingly conceptualized as something separate from personal experience. This is often unseen, but they have to be. For treatment protocols (or mass-marketed workbooks) to exist, which aim to treat the depression or anxiety of thousands of people with the same standardized method, we are stating with little equivocation that the idiosyncratic and personal experience of a given depressed person is independent of their symptoms. While some are critical of this trend because it is dismissive and disrespectful to patients, which it might well be, its most important critique is found in an appeal to critical thought.

Such a critique goes like this. For targeted treatments to stand to reason, those that focus more on "objective symptoms" and less on subjective experience, it would first need to be shown that these things can be theoretically disentangled—that symptoms and idiosyncratic subjectivity are actually different entities that can be dealt with as such. That they can be unravelled from each other is a taken-for-granted assumption on which psychiatric treatment in the modern world rests. But this assumption is faulty. The symptoms people carry are not component pieces of their subjectivity to be individually, extracted, examined, and treated. Symptoms *are* subjectivity, and while it might not seem so, they are formed of the whole of subjectivity. There are not separate subjectivities for depression and health, anxiety and non-anxiety, or anger and calm; therefore, symptoms can never be thought of as a special type of subjectivity, or even elemental parts of subjectivity. Our constructs have become discernable, precisely because there is only one subjectivity marked by experiential shifts. For example, we only know when the thing we call "anxiety" has set in because we know when the thing we call "calm" has not; and we only know depression because we know good spirits.

It is wrong then to assume that symptoms of anxiety are the signal that anxiety has set in. One doesn't know they are anxious because of a special state called, anxiety. Rather, one knows they are anxious because of non-anxiety, because "the rest of subjectivity," though seemingly out of operation, is somehow still present, even if only in memory. If it were not, anxiety would not feel especially important. It would be a subjective state with no meaning every time it cropped up. But it isn't. We notice it as much because of what it is as because of what it isn't. Without contrasting a given experiential state against all others, it would be unrecognizable as a state to begin with. Ironically then, what psychiatry thinks of as a discrete "symptom" is borne of the obvious and undeniable unity of subjectivity. To divide subjectivity into symptomatic and non-symptomatic is off base. It works with words; in experience, however, the two are eternally entangled.

This is precisely the light in which the theoretical failure of the medical model is seen most starkly. Pharmacological treatment, which is often considered the most targeted intervention for symptomatic experience, regularly shows itself in several other kinds of experience—non-targeted ones—in the form of side-effects. If one's mood improves but their sexual drive, vitality, and sense of balance decline, it would appear that unlike in theory, in practice, one's so-called "mood" cannot be isolated from the rest of experience so as to be singly acted upon. Thus, we see that the concept, "mood," might not neatly refer to what we think it does. To the extent that it reaches throughout subjectivity, correlating with non-mood domains, the concept "mood" might refer to *more* than we generally think it does (i.e., if it is entangled with one too many processes from which we normally believe it is distinct). And beyond that scenario, if it reached into enough "non-mood" domains—if it covaried with enough "other" processes—it might drop out as a discrete thing, whatsoever (i.e., it would disappear).

From this lens, atomistic, symptom-reduction models are stripped of all theoretical sense. If subjectivity was as discontinuous and fragmented as they assume, symptoms never could have come into existence to begin with. It's the continuous and fluid state of subjectivity that makes different symptoms identifiable and gives them meaning. If you've ever played with a Rubik's cube, you already know this. Imagine you were looking for the solution, when suddenly, you could see only the blue pieces. The game would no longer make any sense because blue only derives its meaning through the rest of the colors. Thus, symptom alleviation models do not simply undermine and patronize people by separating symptomatology from the life of the person experiencing it; through their attempt to partition "symptoms" from "the rest of experience"—as if these things are quite different—they also quietly yet thoroughly reject reason. Had the makers of the Rubik's cube done the equivalent, they'd surely have no customers.

Overvaluing Language

The symptoms (e.g., anhedonia) and larger constructs they comprise (e.g., depression), in which we are so interested, since they take the form of language, leave something out—something experiential. While this is easy to agree to, conceptually, it's a paradox that earns almost no thought in our field. It doesn't for several reasons, the most obvious of which is that we need language to meaningfully talk about experience. There's no way around this. But when something is talked about for long enough (i.e., experience), the talk and the referent are blurred. What results from our reticence to acknowledge this is a default, field-wide view that our observable and describable symptoms are not just arbitrary markers for experience but meaning-laden entities in themselves.

The implications of this problem are well past astounding, could constitute ten different books, and are routinely and unknowingly disregarded at every clinical turn. As this problem picks up speed, our field becomes not only less interested in experience and thereby less capable of understanding it but rewarded for the capacity to "shorthand it." If it were already on the ropes, this is where our field's interest in contemplating itself is delivered another crushing blow, from which it might never recover. Our value for accurately categorizing human experience is at perfect odds with our value for slowing down to better grasp it, which means we are compromised in our ability to understand it, non-superficially. From this point, we will make less and less sense as a matter of course. The following are three examples of our unfortunate senselessness.

First, consider the well-intended clinician who presents a patient to a treatment team by stating, "Mr. Z has depression." Subsequently, heads nod, which means a consensus about the patient's experience is already developing among the team. But what is being agreed to? This is important to ask because regardless of its relative validity, shared knowledge of some kind is forming. What is consensually known, here? If we know that our constructs are meant to capture experience, that the construct offered (depression) is only a placeholder for experience, and that the treatment team is claiming knowledge of experience, then it can only be concluded that the treatment team is unwittingly populating this construct—depression—with their own experience. Thus, each person's understanding of the patient suddenly becomes based on what this combination and ordering of ten letters—d-e-p-r-e-s-s-i-o-n—means to them.

Isn't this interesting? Somehow, to make sense of symbols that refer to experience (i.e., words), experience must eventually be invoked; otherwise, they remain only symbols. This reveals that even if we conceptualize depression as an external entity that we discovered, marked by symptoms with no necessary relationship to idiosyncratic and personal experience, it cannot possess a single ounce of meaning until we treat it in precisely the opposite manner—until we apply our own experience to it. This is why when the reader sees this word—klxojja—it means nothing (to create it, I punched the keyboard with a few fingers). It is a nonsense word and therefore brings nothing to mind, but if this combination of letters had been used to capture the experience we now call depression, it would mean something (despite that it lacks inherent meaning). Regarding the hypothetical treatment team, all they know of Mr. Z is a product of the often-unchecked reflex wherein diagnostic labels and entire case presentations are imbued with one's own experience. When the next treatment team member meets Mr. Z, whatever they think they know about him, they still only know themselves.

The next and more insidious problem with this kind of language ("Mr. Z *has* depression") is that it has a way of identifying the descriptor as the cause of the problem; that is, "depression" garners explanatory value that it is not logically warranted. Several examples of this phenomenon are easy to imagine. Consider a treatment team meeting in which a patient's symptoms are fully elaborated by one clinician and diagnostic impressions are provided by others. Things might be said like, "she sounds anxious," which brings with it an implicit explanatory edge. Another example would be if Clinician A warned Clinician B that their patient was looking unwell in the waiting room, to which Clinician B responded, "well, he's depressed," as if to say, "here's your explanation." The shared problem with each of these examples is redundancy. Descriptors are stand-ins—and not explanations—for the experiences they summarize. Our ability to attribute depression, *the experience*, to depression, *the descriptor*, is an artifact of language. The clinical problem with this way of thinking is concluding we know something when we do not—when we *could not*.

Consider a patient and therapist dyad that regularly refers to and monitors the patient's "depression," as if it needs to be warded off in order to prevent problems such as social withdrawal and anhedonia. How could this possibly make sense? In effect, they would be tracking things like social withdrawal and anhedonia in order to prevent them from causing things like social withdrawal and anhedonia. Here too, depression has acquired a causal quality. It is thought to be the source of the patient's depressive experience. But does depressive experience cause depressive experience? This is not to say that monitoring depressive symptoms is not helpful in actual clinical work, but we are not doing what we think we are. Something important is happening within this hypothetical dyad, but it isn't important for the reasons we believe.

A final problem with this trend is seen in what it leads to, downstream. The general public, thanks to the zeal with which our field operationalizes human experience, appears particularly taken with characterizing their own subjectivity, and less keen to explore it. This is why people can enter into treatment and, when asked "what brings you in," provide a faithful answer simply by forwarding one or two Diagnostic and Statistical Manual of Mental Disorders (DSM) classics. They could say, "depression." Or, slightly more personalized, "I have depression." If particularly well acquainted with our constructions and conscientious by nature, they might even say something like, "adjustment disorder with a depressed mood," in order to diligently catch us up. Patients genuinely believe that offering us the right diagnostic categories, the right words, provides us with a roadmap for treatment. People want to do us a favor—their therapists—by dismissing the details of their own lives and replacing them with the categories into which their lives fit. This is a sad state of affairs.

Consider what happens, though, when a patient like this seeks treatment only to find a provider who is also quite happy to focus their efforts on identifying and characterizing the problem. Will any attention be paid to what the problem is like? Don't bet on it. For such a treater, the apt label *does in fact* lead to obvious goals and an "indicated" treatment. In cases like this, the patient's subjectivity could garner their own attention and that of the therapist only to the extent that it delivers them to the right "treatment protocol," which was pre-ordained before the patient ever uttered the word, "I."

It's only because of language that we think the presence of a psychiatric disorder causes emergent symptoms; in reality, the presence of the disorder is defined by its symptoms and they are thus equivalent. It's only because of language that we think depression can be treated as a subjective experience unto itself with little relation to the whole of subjectivity; in reality, human subjectivity cannot be partitioned and understood in isolation any more than a puzzle piece can be understood on its own. It's only because of language that when a diagnostic word is spoken, our immediate associations feel like knowledge to us, and not bias; in reality, meaning is put to experiential categories, idiosyncratically, by each person. It's only because of language that upon learning to deftly impact our favored constructs, which we do quite well (e.g., "empirically supported treatments"), we can claim we are changing experience; in reality, the world of constructs is adjacent to the world of experience, and the less this is acknowledged, the more likely we are to thoughtlessly conflate them. To clarify that last point, if I say, "I am depressed," only to say "I am no longer depressed" a few seconds later, my depression has legitimately lifted per the construct world. But in the real world of experience, this sounds ridiculous (because it is).

The operationalization of human experience, while well intended, has corrupted our very ability to think about the human mind. At first, this seems to cause cheapened understandings of important clinical concerns, but our predicament turns out to be much worse than that. Psychology and related fields, which are responsible in the modern world for improving human lives, hold some of the shallowest imaginable views of human life. We don't concern ourselves with the meaning of human suffering, where we might find it, or what we might do with it should we run into it. All such thought is made obsolete by neat and discrete constructs. Currently, we teach our students to help their fellow man by way of the construct world, but the joke is on us, for harm nor healing will be found anywhere but being itself. Our current approach is top-down: we see and label the problem, then we proceed to treat the problem as we have defined it. Such work is, by definition, removed from experience. It has to be. If the problem exists in the experience realm, prior to meeting it there, how could we ever know it?

The most honest and accurate answer is that we cannot. We only think we can because we have gone to such great lengths to taxonomize human life, that we all believe (on some level) that labeling experience is understanding it. This is a preposterous and obscene artifact of language-derived knowledge. Acknowledging it as such is threatening, however, since doing so robs us of all kinds of things. Our know-how, our expertise, and our power are derived from the prevailing method by which we label a problem, sift through all known methods of treating it, identify the most effective one, and then confidently claim it as the solution. At bottom, this process—and the public's faith in it—grants us our expertise. Unfortunately, because we have been sanctioned to write the language of human experience, as if it could be done concisely, reliably, and validly (see the DSM), we have forgotten about its infinite complexity. That is, we have forgotten about reality. I often pose the following thought experiment to my friends who are clinicians in order to keep them honest:

> Imagine it were 6000 years ago, and while our modern-day constructs are yet to exist (e.g., moderate recurrent depression; agoraphobia; paranoia), the experiences they aim to represent do exist. That is, people would experience the states we now call depression, anxiety, and all the rest, but we would have no words for them—and obviously no treatments. Now imagine that someone very troubled comes to talk to you about their life, and they want to feel better. Without our modern constructs what are you left with? What could you do?

This proposition is challenging because it asks someone to consider how they would understand the experience of another, absent the symbols we have made for it. What you would be left with is two minds in relation, wherein one is meant to be of use to the other. But how? How could one mind possibly be useful to another with no method to characterize the subjective experience that has come to harm the person seeking help and no established intervention to treat it? With no constructs to be applied to narratives of experience (i.e., anxiety) nor known methods to influence those constructs (i.e., treatment A), from where would the helper derive any understanding of what has gone wrong for this person or how to help it go right?

In this hypothetical situation, the construct world would be unavailable to be invoked; thus, the helper would quickly realize that the interaction itself has suddenly acquired both more value and different meaning. If narratives about experience, including life history, interactions at work, difficult states of mind, and all the rest could not so quickly generate their accompanying labels, the helper's method of knowing about the patient would shift dramatically. In lieu of our pet words to represent it, the only way to know what experience is like for the other would be to actually come into *experiential contact* with it. That is, the helper would be forced to know the problem by way of the interaction itself. Thus, the here-and-now experience would hold more value than any narrative *about* experience because we would lack the symbolic framework to depict it (diagnostic and experiential descriptors). The encounter itself would become, in the most literal sense, valuable beyond words.

In addition to more value, the interaction would also take on a new meaning. It would shift from a place where human problems are addressed to a place where human problems will manifest; and further, it would morph from a setting bent toward experience derivative (i.e., constructs) to a setting bent toward experience itself. What's even harder to imagine is that absent our language codes for relative difficulty and changes to it (e.g., I am more worried; I am less angry; I'm not anxious), the interaction itself would also be required to mean relative health. I deliberately use the phrase "mean" relative health, and not "assess" relative health, because the latter depends on a distancing from experience and an imperative to code it, options unavailable to us in this hypothetical situation. We would need a way of understanding, in terms of the interaction itself, what exactly improving or worsening quality of experience means. Thus, in this thought experiment, the meaning of the harm, the meaning of the healing action, and the meaning of relative progress would all three be necessarily indicated by way of the dyadic interaction.

The reason this is a thought experiment and not a behavioral one is because it could never happen. Since all language is code for something, we could never operate without symbols that refer to experience, not short of giving up language altogether. Even if we could remove diagnostic terminology from our vocabularies, there would still be the rest of language and the countless ways that it conveys experience in coded terms. However, this only underscores the point I am making. I am inviting the reader to reconsider the meaning of psychotherapy, were experiential problems confined to the realm in which they truly exist—*experience*—and unable to migrate to the language-derived construct realm. In this imaginary world, there would be no language about or references to experience; there would be only experience. In this world, we would be forced to ask a question that our misguided faith in constructs of all kinds affords us the luxury of ignoring: by what method would we understand the experience of another if we acknowledged that language in itself cannot deliver us to it?

An Alternative: Less Verbal Elaboration, More Being

When we place psychological problems firmly in the realm of experience, where they in fact exist, and not in the language we use to describe them, we see that words are not a sufficient vehicle to apprehend them. In turn, this should make us rethink the comfortable feeling of "knowing" that washes over us simply by hearing, applying, or invoking words and concepts meant to capture experience; it should remind us that if symbols and experience are not the same, understanding one does not guarantee understanding of the other; and it should illustrate that as a method of understanding experience, language frankly enchants us in a way that isn't warranted. If we respected the experiential nature of psychological problems, the only information of any value would exist in the form of the present moment because this is the only place experience can ever be apprehended. All else is derivative of what we care about. Thus, the purpose of the thought experiment above is to demonstrate that if we rightly conceptualized psychological problems as experiential in nature, we would soon see that the therapeutic encounter has to mean everything. And not because relational paradigms are in vogue or because we contemporarily understand the power of the interpersonal, but because in the sense I am describing, the therapeutic encounter is all there is.

From this lens, *being with* becomes paramount. But what does this mean? When experience is real and constructs are ghosts, what is the purview of the encounter? Another way of asking this is: if we gave up on both facts about subjectivity (e.g., symptoms indicative of Depression) and our known methods of influencing these facts (e.g., Treatment A for Depression), what would guide us in the interaction? If we keep walking this line of reasoning, we arrive at a place where what we do (and don't do) in any given moment in therapy could only be determined by the moment itself. And if this were true, we could start talking about "best treatment" in the terms it deserves to be talked about. It would no longer refer to the most effective set of known techniques; it would refer to a *way of treating another person* that is in their best interest. Similarly, the concept of knowing changes. "What we know" about the patient's designated and assigned construct takes on trivial significance compared to *the manner in which we know the person sitting across from us.* These conceptualizations of "treatment" and "knowing" warrant supreme importance because they take place in experience, in the air between two people. When rightful primacy is granted to being with, however, things also become more complicated. Why? Because it seems to make us responsible for identifying a method of knowing someone, a way of being with someone, that is most right, given the moment. Yes, it certainly does.

To find such a method, though, a kind of theory needs to be laid out from which the best way of knowing people flows. How else would one know if the best course of action in a given clinical moment is to remain silent, crack a joke, or ask a thought-provoking question? And in a more general way, how would one know what exactly they are attempting to achieve with a given patient over the long-term? To offer such a theory, we need to reclaim the mind; but, to do so, we need to reclaim something of immeasurably greater importance.

Psychotherapy Is Ethics Is Psychotherapy

Whether a clinician working with a patient or a mother talking with her daughter, the manner in which one relates to the distress of another is no fluke. If one prescribes *more realistic thinking*, why do they do so? If one thinks what's needed is a *change of pace*, why do they think so? If one believes *restructuring thoughts* is key, why do they see it that way? If one thinks an *exploration of internal conflict* is in order, why do they think that? Everyone relates to suffering people using their own theories, which look superficially like theories of mind; that is, silent assumptions about the mind appear to account for responses to and prescriptions for distress. Upon closer inspection, though, these theories flow from something more fundamental.

As people encounter other people in psychological pain, their manner as well as their attention is as far from arbitrary as anything could be. What is being offered, as one person aims to help another, is a thinly veiled expression of one's own ethics, one's own philosophy of living, one's own philosophy of life itself. If a father tells his son he needs to work harder in order to feel less depressed, the father betrays a theory not just about the mind but about life, one that ties achievement to wellbeing, perhaps even causally. This is the implicit ethic that accounts for the father's psychological intervention. And we clinicians are no different, not one bit.

The theories we adopt and our consequent way of being with patients flow from the values we hold most dear. An empiricist reading this might claim, contrarily, that no ethics are required to value evidence. Unfortunately, this attitude is the consequence of a mind in arrested development. Are there not ethics that point one at empiricism? And what is evidence, anyway? Are there not assumptions about the world that grant one type of evidence more value than others? Or, what about the empiricist's assumption that with sufficient information about the world, we could fix it? Has evidence not become the means to a broader ethical end related to human progress?

My point is that our preferred ways of thinking about the human mind, including how to best help other minds, are simply reflections of what we find to be important, good, and just in this world. There is not one person who could honestly separate these (and the person who attempts to do so is yet to know themselves). We need to acknowledge this because while not readily apparent to many, if we fail to have ethics, we cannot have the mind, we will cease to exist with any intention or for any purpose, and we will spend all our time in the sterile and meaningless world of construct and intervention.

In a certain sense, then, all that follows might be considered the ethics that drive my understanding of the mind; as a disclaimer though, and a point that betrays my bent, for all of the noise I have made about it, I am only interested in the mind as a matter of consequence. It just so happens to be the only known inlet to the human heart, which is, of course, the real home of ethics, anyway.

Ethics asks you, what do you love? Fairness? Outcomes? The downtrodden? Knowledge? Success? If all theories of mind are theories of ethics, then they are all, at bottom, theories of love. The philosophical veil for my theory of love, which I have tried to describe in this chapter, is this: experience cannot be reduced. We aim to organize it and capture it with words but doing so could never bring us closer to it; nor could it help us to better understand it, not in *its* terms anyway—only in ours, which means, again, we are no closer to it. Experience is the bottom of human psychology and has no constituent parts. Our constructs—depression, anxiety, and hatred, for example—do not exist at the level of experience, despite being used to categorize experience. Yet, prevailingly, this is what we concern ourselves with. We try to treat experience (i.e., actual subjectivity) with constructs (i.e., CBT for Generalized Anxiety Disorder), when the truth is that experience and constructs are of different worlds.

A More Honest Perspective

Efforts to alter experience by way of the construct world are therefore short-sighted. Such attempts are like trying to sweeten the taste of already growing apples by climbing to the top of the tree and pouring sugar all over them. It's too little, too late. Just as there is a process already taking place that will account for the eventual taste of the apples into which superficial sugar will never intervene, so too is experience always already happening. It is always *already here*. We could wonder then why we treat it as if it is an abstraction. It simply isn't one. Unfortunately, in the name of being clever and capable, much of our field can be found swaying in the wind at the top of a ladder out by the apple tree, armed with multiple bags of sugar and the best of intentions. But the ladder is wobbly, and those climbing it seem not to know.

All of our clinical energy is bent toward after-the-fact constructs, toward the ghosts of experience; in turn, we become "knowers" of the highest order. There is little so-called clinical science has not uncovered. However, if we can adopt enough humility to see that experience is the most basic unit of human life and exists outside the grasp of science, verbal sophistication, and cognitive genius, our known methods of working with it have to become less appealing. We realize that helping people with their subjective experience must mean finding a viable way to act more on experience as it stands and less on its derivative constructs. This is how we help people with *their* lives, not merely with *our* constructs.

Moreover, if experience is the most basic unit of human existence, then, logically speaking, the only means we have of improving it is, so too, by way of experience. This is what it means to be the most basic unit. And while it will certainly constitute psychotherapy, in the scheme I am proposing, language needs to be thought of as the most critical means to a more important end: effecting change in experience through experiential impact. What we say to people and what they say to us is critical to psychotherapy, and we could never possibly get away from concepts, abstractions, and constructs, but the most important and profound things in this world must be shown because they exist beyond words and could never be said.

PART II

Wandering About Knowing and Wondering into a Better Method

2

THE MISATTRIBUTION OF KNOWING AND THE SENTIMENT OF EXPERIENCE

There is no Such Floor

The process of knowing—of arriving at, then holding conclusions—is at the very base of all the security we will ever experience. It is grounding like nothing else in that it supplies people with a sense of identity, effectiveness, meaning, and more, all of which makes navigating the world easier. However, there is an often-unnoticed problem in the acquisition of knowledge, one that goes unseen precisely because seeing it clearly would undermine much of the security knowing permits.

It starts out like this. Even if we can readily admit that "knowing" is a needed ingredient in psychological safety, in the realm of experience itself, knowing does not feel *at all* like needing. To the contrary, it feels like the simple acknowledgment of that which is so, true, or real (use whatever descriptor you like—it feels *given*). Think about how strange that is. We do not feel desperate for our knowledge whatsoever, but we must be, for what would we do without it?

That we don't generally feel any discomfort about this paradox simplifies our lives, tremendously. It means we can arrive at this or that conclusion, assimilate it into already existing knowledge, and never again worry about its validity. Over time, that which we now know (but once didn't), comes to feel *even more* given, until our own mind starts looking to each of us like a regular truth warehouse. This state-of-affairs doesn't bode well for a peaceful or examined life, but it comes about for a very simple reason: we are so helped by knowing things, and knowing them clearly, that we are often less than motivated to consider and reconsider all we have come to know or the processes by which we have come to know it. What's more, being unmotivated to practice this kind of introspection means being unskilled in it. Thus, more often than we'd admit, we human beings fall squarely in the "unwilling *and* unable" quadrant of a graph plotting the odds that we might earnestly evaluate all the knowns rolling around our heads.

DOI: 10.4324/9781003305286-5

We simply prefer to not cross examine ourselves. This is no criticism of people because it cannot be. We all need to know. And so, we all do.

However, if we did start examining our own knowledge and the process by which we acquired it, we would see in rather stark terms that we might not know as much as we think we do—even if we need to think we do. We would also see that we might not know for the reasons we think and say we do. Finally, we would gain some insight into why inspecting our own knowledge is so unnatural.

The purpose of this chapter is to do just that—to see more clearly the danger of examining our own knowns; in order to do so, though, we will have to walk right up to the danger. What follows, then, is something like a philosophical exposure therapy.[1] Like all well-intended therapies of this kind, this one is meant to open new possibilities: if we can better grip that from which knowing protects us, perhaps we could begin to see what is required to know anew. This is chapter two's "treatment goal," as it were.

What is Knowing?

What does it mean that if one surveyed the entire world and asked everyone to say everything they "know," while there would be some agreement, the discordance could force a reasonable person to consider whether we share the same world after all? What does it mean that we know different, opposing things? To begin considering these questions, critically, we need to first acknowledge that regardless of the content of the discrepancy, whether over the existence of God or the quality of the Yankees pitching staff, people share one thing, fundamentally, amidst a disagreement: the internal experience of certitude. In this way, both parties do in fact "know," and they would both say so—maybe loudly, at the top of their lungs, and while shaking their respective fists. You might be thinking, perfectly reasonably, that opinions are at stake in such arguments, not actual knowledge, the latter of which is sturdier, backed by proof, and therefore beyond dispute. Underlying this perfectly reasonable view is an assumption that what makes real knowledge real is precisely the fact that it has followed from a real evidence base, found in the real, external world.

What's more, real life seems to prove out this model. Just think of how many times you have discerned *what really is* from *what really isn't* after having found evidence. Ordinary experience shows us the formula, "with sufficient evidence, we can know." More elaborately, "increasing evidence compels us to believe more strongly, and with strong enough evidence, belief crosses over into certitude," at which point we know "for sure." Thus, as we experience it, the connection between evidence and knowing feels white-hot. The two couldn't be more inseparable. After all, how else could we know, how else could we prove what we know, and how else could we persuade another to know what we know but for evidence?

For example, imagine I *show you* that ice turns into water at a certain temperature. Then, I *tell you* that my neighbor turns into a werewolf every spring. You would be more likely to place "ice melts at 32+ degrees" in the category of "things I know," than you would "it would be unwise to visit Rob's neighborhood in April." This is because, on balance, the evidence for my ice claim seems sounder than the evidence for my werewolf claim. You saw the ice melt with your own eyes and the mechanism I'm offering seems plausible, whereas werewolf neighbors are not represented in your existing knowledge structures, and the whole thing sounds completely bizarre (and is).

This example, absurd as it is, shows us an overlooked point about the nature of evidence. It is not some unitary entity that merely by existing provides verification. Instead, it has constituent properties and characteristics which are evaluated together and contribute to its relative attractiveness. This complicates things. The moment attractiveness—*appeal*—becomes one of its characteristics, the very meaning of evidence as usually construed is called into question. Most notably, it implies that we choose it. But evidence is not generally thought to be chosen. To the contrary, we more readily consider it the reluctant and impartial arbiter of *all that is*.

Evidence

Whether spoken in a courtroom, a research lab, or in casual conversation, the word, evidence, brings with it implicit connotations of impartiality, homogeneity, and authority. A mental picture might best reflect this state of affairs. Imagine a cartoon consisting of three or four people with competing ideas, each depicted by one of those speech bubbles. Next to each person's idea are different-sized piles of evidence, depicted by something objective-seeming—maybe piles of science books or Bunsen burners. In the context of all "evidence" signifies in the modern world, the person with the best (i.e., most valid) idea is the one whose associated pile of evidence is tallest. "More evidence equals more true" might be the appropriate adage.

However, if evidence can be more or less attractive, this image is not quite right. It fails to consider that the contents of each person's pile might be differentially weighted—that someone's evidence might *count more*. But who weights evidence? Who determines the "proving power" of each pile's respective contents? And how did everything in the piles become evidence anyway? As a case in point, you might have already concluded that my werewolf claim is so flimsy as to rule itself out as "evidence." It is purely "hearsay" or "gossip," rooted in nothing real. Maybe you've concluded that my neighbor upset me, and now I'm walking around the world, calling him a werewolf to anyone who will listen. "Such antics have no relationship with evidence," you might think. Sure, maybe not. But here we find the base of a much bigger problem. In making a claim about what evidence *is not*, a resulting obligation arises to say what it *is*.

This marks the beginning of a very difficult quandary. As soon as one attempts to define the properties of evidence—to say what constitutes it and what does not—it becomes immediately apparent that doing so requires motivation, like all volitional acts. Yet, the mere presence of motivation calls into question the impartiality thought precisely to define evidence. We cannot construct anything, not a kitchen table nor a definition of evidence, in the absence of motivation. When we make a table, we construct it based on desired ends. We might want it, for example, to seat six, to look half-decent, and to not collapse when guests visit for dinner. And even if it fails on each of those counts, we might hope still that it garners our family's appreciation. Thus, the manner in which we conceive and build it is determined by all of these factors—by the set of things we hope it can achieve. Our conception of the table, but especially the elements we find essential to it, are dictated by the goals we have for it. We are motivated by usefulness, and discerning what is useful from what is not is hardly an arbitrary or value-free process. Nor would we want it to be—it's our table!

In order to know what will make our table useful—*what will make it work in the way we so wish*—we are forced to consult our own goals, which are ultimately the products of personal desire. It is simply not possible to create in the absence of desire. Creation requires volition, which requires desire (or at least will—call it what you want). Whatever we call it, once it is activated, we are moving toward some personal end. The process of creation is inescapably tied to our own goals. Now, this argument could be refuted in a couple of easy ways that miss the point. For example, one could claim that *personal goals* are not required to build a table for *someone else*, a cousin for example. Or it could be argued that some forms of art are explicitly carried out *without preformed goals*, meaning that the creative process does not demand the artist's loyalty to his or her personal sensibilities. But these are semantic points. Making a table for anyone, whether for yourself or your cousin, and making art, with or without a stated goal, is still making. Thus, both acts are still motivated, which means their outcomes are still inseparable from their creator.

When applied to certain things, like tables, what I am putting forth is easy to accept. Of course our personal conception of a kitchen table dictates the manner in which we fashion it. No reasonable person or even an unreasonable person with an ounce of investment in the aesthetic quality of their kitchen would argue this. However, it grates harder on our sensibilities when a similar claim is made about something like evidence. This is because, contemporarily, evidence, along with several related concepts, is thought to be defined by its freedom from the bias of personal sentiment. We tend to think it was formed in a distant land, quarantined from all opinion or ambition, and allowed to develop—a perfect mirror of that which is really so. But neither conceiving of the fundamental characteristics of evidence, the concept, nor favoring one set of evidence over another in day-to-day practice, can be done in the absence of goals. This effectively rules out the possibility that personal sentiment is immaterial to its creation;

moreover, it begins to look like rather essential material. Incidentally, that it is seen as a "value-free authority" (which is itself an oxymoron), seems to account for a growing and paradoxical trend in the modern world, in which a single whisper of "evidence," impartial as it is, inspires more anxious obedience from dutiful bystanders than has any genocidal tyrant in history.

Even good faith uses of evidence, which aim to honestly *show us what is so*, seem to contain a dilemma of logic. Just like our conception of a kitchen table, our conception of evidence must be determined by what it is meant to achieve— what we want from it. What we want from evidence is the ability to discern what is so from what is not. Here is where it gets tricky. In theory, prior to delineating what constitutes evidence, we do not yet have access to what is so and what is not. This is because evidence, which grants such access, has not yet come into existence. Without some idea of what is so and what is not, how then would we endow evidence with the properties that will enable it to actively differentiate what is so from what is not? At least from a logical standpoint, we wouldn't. To accord evidence any "proving power," we must build right into it our already existing ideas of *what is* and *what isn't*. In effect, this is to (even if implicitly) supply the concept of evidence with ends—no differently than our table for six. Yet these ends come necessarily from us, certainly not from evidence, because at the point they entered into the process, evidence was yet to exist (we were still fashioning its meaning).

From this angle, any conception of evidence must rest on a preformed understanding of what is so, an understanding that dictates both what we mean by evidence, and in turn, where it will point us. This is odd when one considers that evidence is meant to be fully free of predetermined aim. Suddenly, we see that this could never be. To claim it could be is to claim that we can construct in the absence of volition—a claim we would never stand for if it was made by the carpenter making our table and charging by the hour. Tables nor evidence construct themselves; thus, tables nor evidence can exist absent goals.

The abstract point I am making is that all conceptions of evidence are inescapably bent in the direction of one's understanding of what evidence might uncover, which is to say, what it ought to uncover, given what one already takes as true with respect to the nature of reality. In seeing this, we also see that conventional wisdom is incomplete. We all believe that evidence accounts for what we know, and in a sense, it does. But it must also be true that some other kind of knowledge accounts for our evidence. This phenomenon appears to least hold in empiricism, modernity's prized method of knowing, but it does hold. It holds for all evidence. We are just reluctant to see it as such.

Observing Empiricism

In a basic sense, empiricism is a method of knowing what is so about the world by way of observation-derived evidence, which reveals relationships between phenomena. At first glance, it seems ludicrous to claim that knowing precedes evidence in this system because conclusions are drawn *after* evidence is evaluated. As one example among thousands, modern vaccines did not exist before researchers identified very specific evidence. That empirical findings follow the evaluation of evidence is not something to be argued with. What can be further considered, however, is all that precedes this process. In line with the discussion above, we might ask, "what was the process by which certain characteristics acquired sufficient favor to mark or constitute evidence—in this case, empirical evidence?"

For all methods of knowing, empiricism and the rest, the meaning of evidence follows from the adoption of certain assumptions. Even if it doesn't appear so—and it doesn't to true believers—empiricism too makes several assumptions. Elaborating all of them is beyond the scope of this chapter, but to make the point, here are a few. First, an assumption is required to know that perception is the most viable path to knowledge, and therefore, that things that cannot be readily observed do not exist (or, at least, are immaterial to understanding reality). Second, that what we perceive with our senses is a true read of the world around us requires an assumption. Finally, the notion that the world is ruled by cause-and-effect relationships, which are readily apprehended by way of human senses manages two assumptions.

Thinking of these and related claims as assumptions is challenging, first of all, for emotional reasons. To suggest that human perception might not be all it's cracked up to be is understandably threatening to humans. We want to believe that our own observations can permit us to know everything that is knowable, and empiricism poses us no pushback—it plays right along, patting us on the back for our well-founded perceptions.

Also, because what science produces contributes to our prosperity, our motivation to tacitly (or hungrily) accept scientific advancement skyrockets, which in turn, obviates any concern, curiosity—and for many people, awareness—about the assumptions that preexist the entire process. Plainly, it doesn't benefit the average person to question the grounds on which science rests because science brings with it so many comforts. However, that the process of science produces powerful medication (e.g., bacteria-killing antibiotics) and the capacity to see what people in other countries had for breakfast (e.g., "Instagram"), does not permit its assumptions a change in status—they are still assumptions. It does mean, however, that the assumptions of science "work" in a way that is of great use to people (in these cases, those stricken with illness that until last century could have killed them, and the ever-growing number of people interested in the waffles of strangers, respectively).

If fear is the first reason we are reluctant to see assumptions as assumptions, conflation is the second. Assumptions are, by their nature, unproven quantities, even those associated with our most revered methods of knowing. Empiricism's assumptions are still conceptions of reality taken as valid *in the absence of proof.*

When looked at honestly, this makes them all the more interesting. In order to understand what they are and how they are decided upon, we have to first think more about their place in knowledge production. What we *do know* is they are the first step. The order of events generally thought to produce knowledge is as follows. First, assumptions are made; then, corresponding evidence is sought, analyzed, and evaluated; and, finally, knowledge is produced. Let's slow down and consider the meaning of the first event, assumption making, as it relates to empiricism.

The Nature of Assumptions

Because the propositions contained in this step (e.g., "reality can be ascertained with perception") are so foundational to the paradigm itself, an unusually honest appraisal would warrant them boatloads more validity than any information the paradigm itself could produce. That is, assumptions underlying the paradigm are so fixed as to have no wiggle room, whereas empirical findings—the products of such assumptions—are always revisable. In fact, this process of revision is how science builds on itself. To see this difference in action, ask yourself which is more certain from an empirical perspective: that the next five days will be partly cloudy (produced by empiricism) or that the best method of predicting weather patterns five days ahead of time involves observation (produced by empiricism's assumptions). While the former can be doubted and its accuracy questioned, if empiricism is to remain intact, the latter cannot. Empirical assumptions, unlike empirical findings, consist of a set of information that is known, known very sturdily, and observation nor anything else holds power to cast upon it any doubt.

This only becomes a problem when it is acknowledged that empiricism, which rests on knowing through observation, knows what it knows most stridently by some other method (incidentally, a method that might be called *faith* in other paradigms). Scientifically oriented readers might take issue with my claim that assumptions represent the staunchest of their claims. They might be more apt to see assumptions as necessary steppingstones to *the real claims*, which are produced by the steps that follow assumption-making. To assuage this reader, let me make two points. First, looking into how empiricism's assumptions are arrived at is *not the same* as refuting them. Secondly, this line of thought is not about empiricism per se; it is about the meaning of assumption across all methods of knowing, across every single form of knowledge, every attempt to know.

For example, this phenomenon might show itself in a debate between a priest and an atheist. The priest might believe that all things of importance cannot be seamlessly observed (assumption), which, along with other things, allows him to *know* of God (assumption-derived knowledge). Similarly, the scientist might believe that human perception best apprehends knowledge (assumption), which means he *does not know* of God, or at least, he cannot rightly conclude whether God exists (assumption-derived knowledge). Without saying anything about who is "right" or "wrong," we can say that neither one of them could possess certitude about their knowledge in the absence of the same certitude for the assumptions on which that knowledge rests. If we accept that assumptions are something different than provable quantities, we start to see something awfully strange, which represents a stride toward danger in our exposure therapy.

While we claim by definition that "knowledge" exists independent of us, whereas things like "opinion" and "belief" do not, it now seems that in order to know anything—whether an empirical fact or a ferocious conviction—we are first required to be highly invested in certain assumptions. We might even need to be *certain* of them, for if we were uncertain, all our "knowns" that follow from them might suddenly feel so flimsy as to prompt us to rename them, "possibles." When this is recognized, the concepts of belief and knowledge, once thought to be qualitatively distinct, are suddenly and eternally entangled, for if we know, we have already believed (whether we can believe it or not).

Paradigmatic Knowing

From this point, incredibly difficult questions follow, questions that are not so much ignored in day-to-day life as never noted. One could ask in good faith, for example, "if all knowledge claims are comprised by some part belief, what is the appropriate breakdown?" Exactly how much belief can occupy a claim before that claim loses its status as "knowledge?" These questions, however, while seemingly logical, betray a much larger problem. Designating a given claim as belief, fact, knowledge, conjecture, or anything else cannot even be done prior to adopting the rules of a particular method of knowing, whether empiricism, rationalism, postmodernism etc. Applying any kind of label (e.g., fact, belief, truth) to any kind of claim (e.g., ice melts at 32+ degrees, my neighbor is a werewolf) can only be done from inside some kind of paradigm, even if only an invisible, implicit one.

Any given paradigm might start with very different ideas than the one next to it. As examples, in religion, knowledge is thought to be derived through methods like faith or revelation, whereas in empiricism, knowledge is derived through observation. In certain branches of philosophy, primacy is granted to reason and logic in uncovering truth, but in postmodern paradigms, logic can quickly lose its standing if it dare elevate anything perennial (which serves also to reveal divergent conceptualizations of reality itself). Moreover, depending on the method by which one knows about ethics, morality might be absolute and unchangeable, or it might be given to us by social processes, including by the historical arrangement of power. Finally, in empiricism, the search for knowledge and the amelioration of human problems are pursuits best taken up in the natural world, whereas religious paradigms might seek both in the sublime.

These are only a few examples, but they show us something strange: the concept of knowledge nor its constituent elements should be thought of as possessing inherent meaning that transcends the whole enterprise of knowing. Rather, knowledge derives its meaning precisely from the rules of a given paradigm and functions precisely according to its preexisting conceptions. Once we see that paradigms are required to know, and that *what counts for what* (e.g., belief *vs.* fact *vs.* truth) is not agreed upon across paradigms, identifying the appropriate makeup of "knowledge" becomes impossible because divergent understandings of what "knowledge is" do not revolve around its ingredients and their ratios.

For example, the difference between rational and empirical knowledge is not that the empiricist uses a heaping tablespoon of sensory information whereas the rationalist uses a pinch, nor is the difference between a postmodernist and empiricist that one simply goes heavier on the "objective truth." The real divergence across these paradigms is much more fundamental than what they contain. There is a more important deviation that precedes the pursuit of formalized knowledge and accounts for variable explanations as to how best pursue it (i.e., it accounts for the variable operations underlying each paradigm's view of knowledge production).

The knowledge of different paradigms (e.g., empirical facts or rational deductions) are generally thought to serve the purpose of describing the world. What is far less thought about, however, is that the underlying operations that result in these descriptors (e.g., fact, deduction, etc.), must *so too* represent claims themselves. While a given claim brings with it an explicit assertion about what is so (i.e., the content of the claim), both the label attached to it (e.g., empirical fact) and the method by which that label was produced (e.g., scientific method) betray a latent but faithful understanding as to how the world is best explained. This is true not just for empiricism. For example, when someone rejects the legitimacy of a claim by calling it "illogical," there is an explicit assertion that the claim is off-base, but there is also an implicit assertion that what would be on-base—what would take more into account *that which is really so*—is a claim that stands up straighter to reason. This means that while verbal descriptors (fact, belief, etc.) function to designate the nature of knowledge claims, they first make their own claims about the nature of the world. Each method of knowing asserts some way by which we would best know, each method self-contained and separate from others, existing in something like its own silo.

The rules and operations comprising a given method of understanding the world, though agreed upon and desirable from within one silo, can lose clout as well as meaning when evaluated by the standards of another silo. What passes for knowledge in one can be relegated to belief in another, and one silo can label a claim "value-free" that would be deemed completely biased by another. This does not mean we cannot know anything, or that all knowledge is of equal value. It only means we cannot know before we adopt a method of knowing. But it also means something even more important than that. While the composition of knowledge is understood differently across paradigms, this divergence, though it manifests in disagreement over classification (e.g., is some given claim, X, true or false?) and in debates between warring silos (e.g., a priest and scientist), originates well before any of this. It originates in the most primordial version of understanding, which preexists all formalized methods of knowing and answers the question, "what is understanding?"

What is Understanding?

It is certainly true that the formalized systems mentioned above have their own rules for understanding the world; and if we asked a representative of each to explain them to us, we would hear some very different things. For example, an empiricist and rationalist might tell us, roughly, that sense perception and cognitive faculties are the basis for understanding reality, respectively. In effect, these propositions (or some similar ones) would constitute the deepest assumptions of their preferred paradigms. From there, we might hear of different human activities (let's say observation and reason, respectively) that yield the right tools (let's say facts and claims gleaned from propositional logic, respectively) for arriving at the most valid view of the world.

The trouble is that nothing stated in the preceding paragraph, by either the rationalist or empiricist, accounts for their respective *arrivals* at their preferred assumptions. In fact, while they have pointed at the source of their preferred paradigm (its assumptions), they have not pointed at the source of their preferred set of assumptions; what's more, pointing at its resultant paradigm doesn't do the trick because the order is wrong (the paradigm grows from the assumptions). Simply put, nothing laid out above elucidates the path by which either person made their way to their respective assumptions in the first place. Thus, asking someone about their preferred assumptions does not betray how they understand. A deeper conception of understanding concerns itself with the process by which people come to their assumptions—those that are, simply, good enough for them.

Unconceptualizable Conceptualizing Apparatus

Every time someone holds in mind a conceptualization as to how the world around them works or has worked, it necessarily takes the form of a proposition—it's the stuff of words and language. However, as part of the path to every conceptualization one could possibly hold in mind, processes were utilized that necessarily defy conceptualization. This means that if one has arrived at a cognitive account, whatever it is, the journey to it required the use of a *vehicle* that itself cannot be arrived at with words.

The Obvious Cases

In certain cases, what I am saying is obvious. For example, imagine being in third grade when the teacher asks the class, "what is 9 x 8?" Suddenly, the image "72" just shows up in our mind, as if it was always lurking there. In hopes of being called on, our hand shoots straight up. We get the question right, and when the teacher asks how we formulated the answer, we throw some multiplication rules at everyone. But it isn't really true that we got there with rules, is it? What's truer about our so-called formulation is that there wasn't one. Somehow, in the very millisecond that the symbol "9 x 8" presented itself, the symbol "72" just clicked into our awareness (when only seconds before, we might have been daydreaming about gym class).

A few minutes later, the teacher asks the class, "what's the best holiday?" Here, we're much more reluctant. But how could this be? While the rules and operations behind the math problem warrant the answer "72" an absolute sense of accuracy, the *lack of rules and operations* behind the holiday question make any answer to it accurate. So, sure, we might be stuck on Christmas versus Halloween, but the truth is that we could name any holiday and still be right (or at least not be wrong). As language goes, it contains no formal rules for finding this answer, but as we see it, the apparent lack of rules does not mean there are none to be followed. What's more, the presence of rules doesn't mean we always trust the answers they furnish. This is why pros and cons lists are notoriously unhelpful: if their yield doesn't do right by some other unsayable factor that has nothing to do with their rules yet *really matters to us*, we crumple them up, deeming them unreliable. The pros and cons list's rules, nor the holiday question's lack thereof have the final say.

Back to the classroom, though. Let's say we eventually land on Christmas, and the teacher asks the follow-up question: "what made you choose Christmas?" Being socialized, we might tell the class that Christmas' gifts trump Halloween's candy, so we ultimately decided on the former. But we have the same problem we had with the math problem. This isn't really true, is it? Over the course of a few split seconds, Christmas just showed itself as the better call. We were just moved to it.

Here is the crucial point. In explaining to the class our arrival at "72" or "Christmas," we have no choice but to utilize language. Thus, whatever we say, it is a depiction, a representation of how we arrived where we did; whatever we say is a conscious calculation *of* our mind *by* our mind, while the *actual* process as it *actually* took place was an activity. More sophisticatedly, we could even attribute the emergence of "72" to something called "short-term memory;" or we could further describe our path to "Christmas!" as one of "realization" or "implicit discernment." In both cases, however, despite moving these processes to the world of representation (by depicting them as concepts), what actually took place can never itself migrate to the world of cognitive representation. In both cases, that being referred to is not really a concept, construct, or representation; rather, it's more like a behavior. This means that no matter what we say *about it*, we are never saying *it*; we are forever referring to it. And what this begins to point at is a strange possibility: subjective experience contains processes that are native to and confined to subjectivity. That is, they themselves cannot make their way to the mind in the form of representation; they themselves can *only be done*.

A Less Obvious Case

To further examine this phenomenon, let's look at another scenario. Imagine being at work and suddenly jumping up, grabbing your keys, and rushing out the door. If someone asked you how you abruptly came to the idea that you needed to hurry, you could say something as simple as "I noticed it was 6 pm and I was late for a dinner reservation." And this is fair enough; it's also true. But what you can't say are the varied attentional, perceptual, and observational processes underlying the experience of "noticing" as you did everything that took place from the time you turned your head to look at the clock you hadn't looked at in three hours, to the time you furiously turned the key in your car. Even if you can lay out the whole course of events in words, the internal processes by which they were mediated will not be found in the representations of them you're offering.

You might feel compelled to liken the internal processes I am describing here to any other kind activity that can *only* be done. For example, if while in the company cafeteria you tell a friend about a new dance you learned at salsa night, you aren't dancing; you're only representing—*and you know so*. The difference with psychic activities is our reluctance to see any of them as representations. Doing so is even unnatural. Because we are with our own minds all the time, feel so familiar with them, and feel so privy to how they work, each of us is fooled into thinking that we have special access to the whole of their behavior—that we can easily and seamlessly capture their innerworkings, fully, no matter what.

What we don't realize—and this is essential—is that, yes, sometimes we are at the salsa lesson doing the actual dance; but sometimes we are in the cafeteria, forever talking *about* something that can only be done—forever *recounting* some process of mind, not *doing* it. My point here is that we tend to take these things as the same, even though they aren't. There are at least two reasons for this mistake. One has to do with proximity. Because we are *always* in our minds (and only *sometimes* at a dance lesson), and because our minds are *always* doing something, our primary relationship with our minds is one of action. In turn, we conflate, for example, the doing of attention with the representing of attention that would take place if someone asked, "how'd you notice that?" Basically, we forget that the explanation does not mimic the process, or more to the point, that the explanation *isn't* the process. In contrast, we'd never make this mistake when recounting our salsa dance. We know what's dancing and what's talking about dancing; and even more importantly, there is no world in which they seem remotely similar. The next and related reason we conflate the *doing* of mental processes with the *thinking* and *saying* of them has to do with language. Because we are saturated in our own use of language, and because it seems to capture the events of the external world pretty well, we assume that with the proper use of language, every one of our mind-housed products—every conceptualization and formulation we hold in mind—can be faithfully accounted for.

But we are wrong about all of this. All that we come to hold in mind (e.g., "I better leave or else I'll be late!") is derived with internal processes that can never be said and can only be done (e.g., observation, attention, perception). Therefore, any after the fact explanation as to how exactly we conceptualized or formulated this or that is *incomplete* to the extent that language merely *represents* activities that not only happened but of which we were *entirely unaware* as they did. This is why telling someone "how we noticed X" is not the *real* how; it is forever a representation of the *actual* activity by which we *actually* perceived X. This is despite that we never naturally distinguish the two. As far as we are concerned, our after the fact story of how we perceived *simply is* how we perceived.

Implications

The next question is to ask what would happen if we admitted that subjectivity contains processes to which we can give names and talk about, but that, *themselves*, we can only ever do (e.g., attention, perception, observation). Probably what we would try to do next is observe them; with our verbally sophisticated minds, we would try to make more sense of them. For example, let's say I decided that it is important for me to devote some thought to the nature of my attention, or to slow down and better examine the quality of my perception and observation in the social world? And let's say in doing so, I arrived at some pretty good ideas as to how my attention and perception move throughout the interpersonal landscape. These would be good outcomes. Yet, while they might move me closer to *something*, they don't capture an account of my attentional and perceptual style as seamlessly as I think they do.

We know this because, first of all, the data yielded by these pursuits, "information about the movements of my attention and perception," necessarily take the form of conceptualizations. This means that *neither do they* contain within them all the different processes that created them—the same ones I was trying to track. Thus, something is still missing. What's more, would it have been possible for me to observe my attention without attending? Or to examine the nature of my perception without perceiving? Just so you know, my claim is not that this kind of self-observation isn't useful; rather, I'm claiming that gaining an "understanding" of these unsayable—only doable—processes, those that are native to subjectivity, requires that we put them to use (assuming an "understanding" *is* a conceptualization). Any formulation as to how these exclusively doable processes work must have relied on them, which further shows that their true form is in *being carried out* (not represented). As shown here, even when we try to put them in some other form (i.e., a concept to be examined), we fall short, for we were first required to activate them in order to do so.

This shows us again that there is something contained in our path to formulations and conceptualizations that is only ever an activity; and further, that regardless of the verbal understanding we hold in mind as to *how* we have arrived at this or that formulation, there is always *something else* that has moved us to it—something we can never capture because *having captured something* is the very signature of this "something else." Thus, whatever this "unconceptualizable thing" is, we cannot have formulations that are not informed by it, nor can we have conceptualizations that were not run through it. All of this is to say that there is some apparatus forever confined to being—and never found in representation—that contributes to all we have represented, formulated, and conceptualized. What's more, while every conceptualization we utter has inevitably been generated *by it*, at least in part, not a single one of them has *expressed it*, as it cannot be expressed.

In this light, let's return to our rationalist and empiricist. When we left them, they were trying to prove the superiority of their respective assumptions. But now we see that calling them "assumptions" or "first principles" in no way makes them the beginning of how they understand, even if their respective paradigms of understanding grow from them. Their statable assumptions are the culmination of a conceptualizing process that is confined to their respective subjectivities. Sure, the way the empiricist and rationalist understand the world is different. But it isn't different because the assumptions to which they subscribe are different; rather, the assumptions to which they subscribe are different because the way they understand the world is different. Particularly, something in the apparatus that produces their conceptualizations is different, which accounts for their divergent manners of formulating (i.e., an activity) and its divergent yields (i.e., expressly stable propositions). And we can call the yield "assumptions," but they are not known with hesitation or reluctance of any kind because despite being born of a process that refuses articulation, it is a very personal process, nonetheless.

What's more, so-called "assumptions" or "first principles" are only argued over because they so happen to be the deepest difference that can be said. In fact, an argument like this *is* the language-situated manifestation of a difference that both preexists language and has moved both parties to theirs, but which language cannot capture. That is, in a debate between an empiricist and rationalist over the merits of their systems, words are not capturing but working on behalf of the real difference. The real difference, the manner by which they were driven to the conceptualizations they now hold and about which they disagree, cannot be argued over because it cannot be thought nor said. It can only be done. And in ordinary, day-to-day life, as in a debate like this, if we possess formulated thoughts and words, something so too has already been done.

Unconceptualizable *and Idiosyncratic* Conceptualizing Apparatus

The phenomenon laid out above is essential to the rest of this book because it is essential to human life. We are ruled by our way of *doing* conceptualizing; we are ruled by the act of it, which our cognition is less equipped to trace and understand than we believe. Though we don't always see it, in the same way we are sometimes only depicting a newly learned salsa dance, we are sometimes only depicting the course by which we arrived at some formulation of the world. Here is an example.

Imagine, hypothetically, that two people experience the same exact event: being given the wrong change at a café. In response, Tom lands on the formulation, "the cashier tried to swindle me," whereas John lands on, "the cashier made a mistake." The two conceptualize an *identical situation* differently. And so, we might even begin to say that the conceptualizing apparatus confined to subjectivity, which *is* or *fuels* or *is attached to* one's manner of conceptualizing, is different for Tom than for John. Whatever it is, it has different properties. There is something idiosyncratic to it.

Now imagine talking to Tom and John after their encounter with the barista. If we asked them to explain how they arrived at their respective formulations, they could. Tom might tell us that he noticed the cashier giving him a dirty look prior to the interaction; or he might tell us that devious people always peg him as an easy target. On the other hand, John might tell us that he didn't notice any foul play whatsoever, or he might even sympathize with the cashier, hinting that she seemed tired or stressed out. In light of the current discussion, however, what are these follow-up explanations? Better yet, what aren't they? Well, they certainly aren't made from the same substance that aided Tom and John in arriving at their original conceptualizations in the first place—they couldn't possibly be, since the explanations they are now offering exist in the form of language.

Neither Tom nor John is offering the cause of their original conceptualization. Instead, both are offering further expressions of it, further renderings of it. Despite taking a different form (i.e., "the cashier was looking at me funny") than the original conceptualization (i.e., "the cashier tried to rip me off"), nothing said is a description of the trip to the first conceptualization; it is only a description of the view, once landed. This is why, sorry to mix examples, the most accurate answer to our teacher's question—*"how* did you land on Christmas?"—is silence, for anything we could possibly say is only more evidence *that* we've landed there.

All that is represented in Tom's mind, from the original proposition (e.g., the cashier swindled me) to every supporting piece of evidence he names (e.g., the cashier gave me a dirty look when I ordered), overruns the mark. They are not *causes of* but *testaments to* how he understood. The deepest things we can name, since they can be named, are still not the truest causes of any conceptualization or formulation to which we have come; rather, they are consequences of the real cause, which defies language, conceptualization, and representation. Thus, even if Tom can look for, identify, and say the deepest verbal assumption on which all his interpretations rest (e.g., "I am mistrustful"), this too is the yield of something he cannot say. Even if he is aiming to, he still isn't saying what makes him different from John because the real difference is something native to subjectivity, something that never exits subjectivity. It is forever contained there. By this, I mean that it is never accessible with thought because in order to think toward it, as if it were a concept divorced from him, he would be required to use it (we all would).

The Inevitable Misattribution of Knowing

As this unconceptualizable apparatus goes, we can only ever say what has come from it, never what has gone into it; everything we think and say are its products, not its ingredients. Ultimately, any answer to the question, "why did you see it that way," is in the *deepest* sense (not in the *commonsense* sense), only more evidence of *having* seen it that way. This is most plain in people who often explain variable situations in the most unvarying of ways. For example, someone who is always seeing cynically, always observing cheaters and liars, gives the impression that the *real why* of their formulations is buried underneath all their *stated whys*; they give the impression that there is something more than what they say, which accounts for how they have understood. And this is absolutely true. The real why is embedded in—or *just simply is*—the very way they see, and not in the way they explain what they've seen. This is where the *real why* is for all of us.

Here is what this might mean in terms of practical life. We might know that our coworker was fired because our boss feels threatened by him, or that our poor grade on an exam was due to our decision to drink bourbon instead of study, or that our good luck surfaced as a cosmic reward for our ethical behavior. Yet, what's *more real, more true, more fundamental* than any of these formulations is that something native and confined to our own subjectivity has catalyzed them, has driven them, and rests underneath them; what's more, it is something to which we are blind since it something from which we are never removed. It's something that is always there, attached to our perception, observation, and thought, accounting for each—and it isn't a thing at all.

My point is not to tear down the utility of objectivity or to promote perfect skepticism but to instantiate one of this book's most central themes: that which we grip in our conscious minds and call "assumptions," on which the thing we call "evidence" rests, is not what we most deeply know, even if it is the deepest thing we can find in cognition. Somehow, we already know things, which have steered us to our consciously held knowns. This causes a fundamental complication in knowing: the inevitable misattribution *of* knowing. Through the natural course of thinking, we misattribute what we consciously hold in our minds as "so." This is because in attributing, we must defer to the rationales that constitute language-based explanations. In turn, we necessarily pass something over, something we can never find in mind. The upshot of seeing this means seeing something very strange about knowing.

Completing the Exposure Therapy: There is no Such Floor

An honest and courageous journey into one's own mind, aimed at turning up the ground floor on which all of one's conscious knowns rest, reveals the oddest thing and concludes our exposure therapy: no such thing will be found in mind.

There is no such floor. When taken seriously, this yields what is perhaps, at once, the most humbling and threatening perspective a person can hold with regard to their own knowledge, since it removes the power one usually grants one's own mind to account for itself. In short, one cannot know exactly how their knowns developed, since attempts at knowing such a thing requires the process of conceptualization, the yield of which would not capture but would instead rely on what it seeks (since anything we can know enough to say, explanations for our "knowns" included, maintains developmental origins, all of which we cannot say). From this viewpoint, all our justifications, explanations, and proofs for knowing what we know miss the boat, as they are necessarily constructed from experience as *represented* (i.e., cognition), whereas our knowns themselves emerge from processes confined to experience itself, processes that themselves refuse to be represented. This isn't to say that we can't think *about* that which makes us think how we do; it's just that we can't *think* that which makes us think how we do.

From this perspective, it first appears that in order to better grip the source of our knowns, we would have to better understand this informulable, unconceptualizable coefficient of subjectivity. But not so fast. Because understanding ends in some formulated idea, anything we could "understand about it" is forever its consequence—as opposed to *it itself.* The alternative, then, is to apprehend, while in action, that which moves our mind in the way it so moves. This is not the kind of apprehension to which we can think or say ourselves. In fact, to get there, we shouldn't be thinking or saying at all. We must stop talking, stop thinking, and go inward, into experience. It is only there, not in the external world nor in our formulations or conceptualizations—all of which are concepts to which we misattribute all we know—that we will find the true root of all we know. It will wash over us in being, in the form of *this-ness*, not conception of this, in the form of *sentiment*, not words.

Knowing Anew

To know ourselves, we must find that which simultaneously rules and evades our minds. And to change someone, whether self or other, something in *the way* one comes to know (i.e., the way one conceptualizes and formulates) must change. This is in blunt contrast to changing the details of that which one *does* know (i.e., their resultant, mind-housed conceptualizations), or changing *how one understands* how they understand. Real change is in the changing of how one *does understanding*—nothing else. For this, something must change within the domain that cannot be said or thought, not within the domain of its fruit—everything that can be. The only real change is change that happens here. Because it is in the simple, inarticulable sentiment of experience that knowns are made, it is within the simple, inarticulable sentiment of experience that all the therapeutic action lies.

Note

1 For non-clinical readers, an "exposure therapy" is a type of psychological treatment in which patients are progressively exposed to a feared stimulus (e.g., a snake, a bridge, or even certain memories), ultimately making it more tolerable. As this chapter goes, what I hope to make more bearable is the unthinkable.

3

THE STRIVING MIND

Knowing in the social world is nothing if not variable. Imagine finding ten people who have known Emily in different capacities, at different points in her life, and with different levels of intimacy. What would happen if you asked each of them, "who is Emily?" Given the variability of their answers, you might find yourself shocked that all ten are talking about the same person. Moreover, how would you know which person is "most accurate?" The one who has known her the longest? The one with the least motivation to see her through rose-tinted glasses? Or maybe "accuracy" is the average of all ten responses? The key here is to notice that one's own perception of any given thing (in this case, a person) is a tiny drop in an ocean of perceptions of that very same thing.

And what exactly are the interpretations that follow from one's own perception? An honest inquiry into how we derive them reveals that all they require of us is a feeling that we are sure, not proof that we are right. Think of that: knowing in the social world (i.e., landing on certain conclusions) can happen in the complete absence of accuracy. While it is true that more reflective, thoughtful people tend to be more attuned to times when they got swept up into some conclusion about which they could not really be sure, being "sure" of things without reason is an inclination for most people (maybe all people, to some degree).

Thus, *some of the things* on which we have landed and deemed "true of the social world" are true; but *all of the things* on which we have landed and deemed "true of the social world" are felt to be true. At bottom, each person's universe of consciously held knowns is not simply the category of ideas on which their perception and thought have landed but on which these processes have landed *and stuck*, the only necessary adhesive for which was one's very own conviction. If we have any hope of understanding people, including ourselves, we must see that we are invested in how we see. This is the sole path to seeing more.

DOI: 10.4324/9781003305286-6

One way to start thinking about the personal investment required to "know" is to consider what is most undeniable about any piece of knowledge one could possibly hold in mind. Naturally, we might take the *content* of our own knowledge (and implicitly, its validity) to be its most indisputable feature, but it turns out that its validity is quite easily denied simply by rejecting the assumptions on which it rests; and while *we* wouldn't reject our own assumptions, *others* certainly might. For example, if I'm no fan of the death penalty because I believe in the sanctity of human life, what happens if I find myself talking with someone who sees human beings as just another animal, bound only by the rules of the jungle? It's not that my argument is less sound than usual in this person's company; it's that its soundness doesn't matter, not when underlying assumptions vary so much. Thus, not only is validity not the marking attribute of our knowns; it fails to be a meaningful concept in the absence of shared assumptions.

On the other hand, a feature of one's own knowledge that cannot be denied is the fact of one's involvement in its development. As discussed last chapter, one's own input is a coefficient, an inevitable appendage, of anything one holds as so; after all, arriving at certain knowns required an arriver. At first, this idea seems merely to mean that human input is essential to the *pursuit* of uncovering reality. However, when any reality we could ever find is the product of our pursuit to find it, this view goes not far enough. Arguably, the pursuit of reality is not all that is marked by one's own input; so too is anything this pursuit yields, anything one might point to and call *reality itself*.

In this light, human contribution threatens to represent a more innate characteristic of reality than any depiction of reality it could produce, which means we all ought to think harder about all we take as real. The knowledge we arrive at, which we think captures reality "as it really is," is brought to bear by a more native, inescapable, and arguably more essential element of reality. If we want to understand the social world in which we live, we must understand it as the world we have assembled, for the social world is made of our own striving.

The Striving of Behavior

Because human action is both goal-oriented and largely under the control of the actor, our default view of "striving" is to see it as the principal feature of behavior. This is an easily understandable perspective, given that our action so readily impacts the environment, so often in just the way we wish. For example, when we brake, we slow down; when we study more, we get better grades; and when we ask for the salt, it makes its way to us. While we couldn't possibly be wrong about any of this, our decided and apparent effect on the world around us ends up creating a hole in our explanatory style. In particular, we become far too attuned to our behavioral striving as a means of explaining ourselves, only rarely seeing that human striving is constituted in more than mere action.

Misunderstanding Motivation: Paradigms of Impact

Let's assume that every weeknight at 8 pm, I find a book and read for two hours. This course of events highlights the most obvious characteristics of striving. It is planned, effortful, and behavioral in nature. However, in attending to these properties first and foremost—and we all do, naturally—we begin to *account for our behavior* through a "paradigm of impact." We believe that we do A (search for the book) in order to achieve B (read). Owing to our ever-impending plans to impact the world around us, this model of explaining our behavior seems valid and reflective of reality in almost any moment we exist; on another hand, though, it comes to pose incredible problems to self-understanding. Because we are so accustomed to acting out behavior chains like this one, misunderstanding ensues: we begin to locate the motivation for our behavior in *the external world*. In casting ourselves as the sum of our action, we begin to feel that we do things for their external effect—and, yes, we do.

But when too focused on the *impact* of our action, the whole enterprise of acting in the world appears fundamentally effect driven, even to the actor. That is, actors account for a given act in terms of its intended outcome (i.e., that which it aims to achieve), as opposed to its origin (i.e., the internal factors that induced it). This produces in people a damaging conflation: the *target* of one's motivation is often mistaken as its *source*, resulting in disastrously superficial views of both self and other.

Example 1

Here is an ordinary example. Imagine Person A asks Person B why they are going shopping, to which Person B responds, "because there is a sale." In effect, Person B is offloading their own motivation, their own agency, to whoever works at Macy's and decided today was a good day to make things 20% cheaper than usual. To whatever extent Person B's explanation sounds like a viable reason as to why any one of Macy's 300 shoppers would be there on that day, it fails to be an explanation of themselves.

At bottom, the problem I am describing is one in which we human beings fail to recognize that our own motivation, our own desire—or at least, *ourselves*—is an ingredient in all our behavior. For any action to be taken, no matter how trivial, there must be an actor; and for actors to act, there must also be an internal impetus. But because we in modern life are not oriented to the internal, much of our behavior *appears to us* as dictated by something external (e.g., "what do you mean *why* am I going shopping? I already told you: there's a sale!"). This example shows us precisely how we lose track of ourselves. The shopper reveals that, as far as she knows, nothing internal to her was required for her to become motivated to go shopping; implicitly, this also means that she believes she became motivated to go shopping in the absence of her own volition. While this example might seem trivial, keep your eye on its psychic implications: without seeing the voli-tion *in* one's own behavior, how could one ever find the motivation *behind* it? Of course, one couldn't, which makes one's prospect of locating themselves amid all their action in the world vanishingly small.

Example 2

Imagine it is some weeknight in June and I am looking for my remote control because I want to watch the Yankees game that starts in a few minutes. At the very same moment, my neighbor knocks on the door to ask me if I drove over his potted plant with my car. But before getting to that, he sees me shuffling things around and says, "What are you doing in here?" I respond, "I'm trying to find the remote because the Yankees are on in five minutes." He accepts this answer and proceeds to politely accuse me of running over his plant.

Now imagine the same situation, except in this scenario my neighbor turns up at my door, only to see me tearing my living room apart. Let me set the scene. There are feathers from destroyed pillows floating about the room; pictures are off-center; I appear to be in a manic fit of agitation; and I'm sweating profusely. I finally hear the doorbell on the fifth ring and proceed to answer the door, look-ing disheveled and distraught, as if I had just sprinted 12 miles. Upon greeting him, my neighbor says, "What are you doing in here?" I respond, "I'm trying to find the remote because the Yankees are on in five minutes."

In both scenarios one and two, I truthfully told him my aim: I was doing all I could to find the remote in order to watch the Yankees. In the first scenario, where I was not violently flailing around while doing so, he seamlessly accepts my explanation—it suffices. In the second scenario, however, it probably wouldn't work like that, and we must see why. Sure, I have told him what I am hoping to achieve—my goals as it were—but this answer does not satisfy him. In response, he could very easily say, "Right, I see that, Rob. But what are you *doing*? Seriously, what the hell is going on with you? It looks like a tornado went through your living room and you look like you've been running laps in here since noon." In this case, hearing of my behavioral goals for impacting the environment (i.e., turning on the game) does not satisfy him. He is asking me what I am doing, now keen to the fact that a *better explanation* would involve pointing at myself, as opposed to—or at least, in addition to—pointing at my television.

Now, here is the incredibly interesting point. While it is always true, and in fact, can never *not be true* that all volition requires an actor, we only see it as such, selectively. What I mean is that we are genuinely blind to it. This is evident in the first scenario as my neighbor, with no good reason not to, simply accepts as an explanation for my motivation, its target. He didn't say, "I know your plan is to watch the Yankees, Rob. What I was asking is what *about you* motivates you to watch this baseball game right now, as opposed to drive to the store and buy ice-cream, plan a trip to the Swiss Alps, or do your laundry." He could have though because some internal impetus prompted me to do what I am doing, to the exclusion of doing anything else.

The moment we acknowledge that existing itself is defined by a series of inescapable decisions to do A (not B), and X (not Y), we see that even the most passive of behaviors require of us input and volition—even if only the amount required to not do something else. Behavior requires an agent; and for any given behavior, alternatives abound. This might seem so obvious as to be unnecessary even to mention; despite its obviousness, though, it is routinely off our radars, the major consequence of which is that we are misled into an illusion. Many people walk around life believing, even if only implicitly, that the presence or absence of internal motivation is dependent on the act—that some things require motivation and others don't. This ethos is bad for us, yes, because it keeps us from knowing of our responsibility for all of our behavior, but also because it alienates us from ourselves. It prevents us from seeing ourselves fully, which we must do, not just for the sake of our conduct but for the sake of our souls: seeing more of oneself is always a gift.

Thus, without a compelling reason not to, we misplace motivation. We often fail to separate its source from its target, thereby locating the roots of motivation in the world and not in ourselves. While this way of thinking is somewhat natural, it blinds us to ourselves. The notion that we "do A in order to achieve B" is too well-learned and obstructs us from self-understanding. Once instantiated, this way of thinking renders us unable to recognize the impetus within. It also happens to make little logical sense, which I will quickly explain here.

Desire is Not Near but Here and Everywhere

In the most ordinary sense, we could say that my motivation for making coffee (A) is drinking coffee (B); however, this perspective misses the spirit of motivated behavior (which is all behavior). That B follows A in the observable world might mean that A caused B. For example, you could say that the outcome, a pot of hot coffee sitting in my kitchen, was *caused by* a whole course of steps that preceded its presence (e.g., buying coffee, grinding it, etc.). In a sense, this is beyond dispute.

However, even if one caused the other, one need not have motivated the other. As strange as it sounds, the tangible outcome, a pot of coffee, is not what motivated my quest to make it. As motivation goes, the quest and the outcome are better thought of as a single unit, motivated by something else entirely. Applied to this case, I am not motivated to make coffee by the prospect of drinking coffee; rather, I am motivated to *both* make and drink coffee by *my love of coffee.*

For most people, only when it becomes especially evident that a given actor has a very personal stake in generating some desired effect, do they move away from effect-oriented explanations of behavior. Recall my neighbor, who does not construe me as a motivated agent until I behave bizarrely, at which point he is hit over the head with the fact that my behavior is more about me than any mid-season Yankee game. In effect, he is saying: "what's *really* driving your behavior? *And don't say the external world!*" However, effect-oriented explanations should *never pass* in explaining motivation. Every instance in which the motivation for some behavior is pinned on its intended effect leaves something out. It tells us that we execute behaviors A (buying coffee), B (grinding it), and C (pouring boiling water through it) in order to achieve effect D (consuming 2+ cups of coffee before 7 am), but it fails to explain the emergence of D. That is, this model fails to account for the materialization of the desired effect (i.e., *why D?*).

You see, whatever has motivated the goal of drinking coffee has also motivated the process of making it; and whatever has motivated the goal of watching the Yankees has also motivated the search for the remote. Finding the motivation for some behavior in its intended effect, while commonsensical, wrongly separates the motivation for that behavior from the motivation for its effect. They are usually one. Thus, the *real* task of understanding any behavioral sequence is understanding what has made its intended effect desirable. "Paradigms of impact" account for the way we intend to influence the world but provide us no tools for explaining why we intend to influence it in the way we do. Sure, I am searching for a remote in order to watch television, but how and when did watching the Yankees become a desirable goal?

Maybe the reader finds all of these ideas so obvious and digestible as to be wondering why I have spent so much time laying them out. But this might be due to the fact that they have been presented in the form of inconsequential abstraction and trivial examples—shopping, coffee, and baseball games. My point is to show that *any time* one has acted, which in all its forms is inherently achievement-oriented, one's own motivation was required. In the absence of self-examination, though, this truism is very easy to miss. To reincorporate it, one would be required, while looking at all of their behavior, to also look boldly at the fact of its *appeal*. This is a practice not for the faint of heart. It assumes that the behavior we engage, at least when compared with that we do not, is *attractive* to the actor. At first, this might sound like a recipe for an extremely harsh vision of personal accountability, but it isn't for one reason. Our behavior, all of which we must be motivated to carry out, not only *need not* be good, virtuous, or helpful to us; we *need not* even consciously approve of it. It need only appear to us as a prospect with enough viability to be followed. But why does it?

A Deeper Striving: That of Mind

To answer this question, we must first see that thought produces certain conceptions and not others, which casts cognition as a discriminating process. In thinking, we land on *these* goals, conclusions, and rationales—which ignite corresponding action—not *those* ones. Thus, while behavioral striving is a result of goal-conception (i.e., we do things after deciding to), a more fundamental kind of striving results in the production of goals—and more broadly, in *cognitive production*, generally.

Our cognitive destinations (e.g., propositions, decisions, rationales) might be perfectly well-thought out, and even beyond criticism. But this cannot change the fact that one's journey to them required one's own attention, perception, and thought—one's own cognitive volition. Compared to where we usually see it, this acknowledgment moves up *preference* in the process of mental activity: naturally, we see it reflected in where a given cognitive path has led, but upon closer inspection, the path itself must have been made of preference. In fact, the cognitive process resulting in our arrival at this or that "known" could not have even gotten off the ground, let alone led anywhere, without the thinker's energy and volition. From this angle, something very interesting about the nature of thought comes into focus. We don't just want our consciously held conclusions (which move us to our behavior); in a deeper sense, we also want our way to wanting them, though we don't always see this or feel happy to agree to it. As for our arrival at this or that cognitive destination, we prefer to pin the trip on things like reason, rationality, and good sense.

Being sensible, we can often acknowledge that constituted in our own ideas, perspectives, and interpretations is personal input, even desire—after all, it is us who arrived at them; but even so, experientially, somehow, we are often out of touch with the desire that must be embedded in the cognition that transports us to them. This is because our cognitive products (e.g., conclusions, rationales) are produced by processes that, from within subjectivity, do not feel borne of desire. As examples, desire doesn't seem to be a player in one's rationale to buy a crib when a new baby is on the way, nor does personal input seem to be involved when one grabs their coat before leaving the house in a snowstorm. If we're honest, it feels like both courses of action, which the thinker conceived then followed, *produced themselves* as the necessary solutions to the problems at hand. But can courses of action, as if endowed with their own volition, somehow present themselves to us? No; as our attention, perception, and cognition flit around the external world, generating a hierarchy of viable goals, plans, and rationales, there is a force embedded within them, a kind of *force for preference*, that makes certain conceptions—and not others—accessible, viable, followable.

To account for our motivation, then, we must dig deeper. Not only are we wrong to find the motivation for a given behavior in its intended effect (i.e., a paradigm of impact); we are also not quite right to find the motivation for a given behavior in the thought that preceded it and made it viable. All of the behavior in which we are engaged, which seems motivated by the thought that preceded it, is actually more motivated by that which motivates thought, causing it to land where it does: some force for preference.

At first blush, this view seems to cast the whole of thought, both *what it yields* and *the process by which it yields*, as desirous; after all, it is made of partiality, proclivity, preference. In effect, this is true. However, where desire means conscious wanting, calling thought "desirous" is somehow unfair to the thinker because whatever moves thought must exist outside of thought, which means whatever moves thought is something of which *thinking itself* cannot make the thinker aware; thus, thought is, yes, motivated by something, some force for preference, but the thinker need not be privy to it.

This doesn't mean that we aren't fully responsible for all the conceptions we produce, or for every behavior that follows from them. We are. But it does reveal why we are apt to locate our reasons for some conception (i.e., some decision, plan, or conclusion) before locating the motivational force behind those reasons: because, in a sense, we can't. Despite reigning over the movement and destinations of conscious minds, as it isn't *of* conscious mind, this very force isn't *traceable* with conscious mind. Stranger still, this would mean that despite housing them, our conscious minds need not necessarily *want* its conceptions, even if some other part of us certainly does (i.e., the unthinkable force for preference by which our minds have been moved to them).

Thought in the Social World

While our explanations for our own behavior and that of others aim, by definition, to explain the world, from the vantage point suggested above, we can now see that they themselves must reflect preference, since they are products of thought. This is especially true of our interpretations in the social world. As day-to-day examples, firmness in speech might be read as characterological arrogance by one person but as confidence by another; old friends might disagree as to whether it was interaction A or B that caused the recent strain in their relationship; one employee might see their boss rolling her eyes at a subordinate and deem her a tyrant whereas another employee might see her as authentic or non-coddling. Whatever one's conclusion, one couldn't have drawn it without one's own input.

What's important to see is that we draw conclusions by way of criteria that we produce, which then dictate our understanding. Each of us has preset ideas that we bring to—and do not derive from—interpersonal life, which we follow and utilize in order to understand. For the employee mentioned above, watching his boss rolling her eyes has made her a "tyrant." While he might feel he has aptly characterized his boss' soul, what is most indisputable here is not whether the boss is a tyrant, or even what tyrant means to him; rather, what's most indisputable is that *he has interpreted tyranny*. From this view, it is easy to see why "explanations of the social world" (a phrase that itself implies prioritization of accuracy) are all of them, arguably, circular. It is *we* who set the criteria for our own constructs (e.g., tyrant), and it is *we* who identify when these criteria have been satisfied (e.g., eye-rolling authority). And when they are, we point to the world as if it fulfilled our criteria. We must be wrong, though. The world, while known to provide events, is less prone to providing interpretations. In fact, it's never provided one.

From within subjectivity, it seems that we have explanations and interpretations of the social world in order to explain and interpret the social world. This story is bolstered by the timing of things: holding explanations follows from seeking and creating them. Yet, *the goal of having explanations* does not motivate *the act of explaining* any more than the *goal of drinking coffee* motivates the act of *making coffee*. Just as a third variable, desire, motivates *both* the making and the drinking of coffee, so does it motivate *both* the seeking and the holding of explanations. While we set out to explain the social world in order to have explanations, we would never do so if doing so was not a valuable state of affairs; and having explanations is valuable, only not for the reasons we think.

Our story about our explanations of the world is that they are helpful because it is helpful to be accurate about the world. But in the context of the discussion so far, this doesn't really hold water. Moreover, consider the range of conclusions that people draw from the social world. We arrive at very different interpretations about the very same things, and any given one can satisfactorily "explain" for a given person. This confirms that having an explanation is not serving the purpose of being *accurate*, at least not in some objective sense, however that might be measured. When an event can be interpreted or explained in as many ways as there were witnesses, something other than "seeing things as they are" must be behind each person's perceptual and cognitive striving (this also assumes "as they are" is one thing). If not by way of their accuracy, which is the low hanging fruit we settle for, how do particular *products of cognition* (e.g., particular conclusions, rationales, and explanations) come to garner value?

Having an Understanding vs. Understanding

Before the purpose of thought is to understand the social world, it is to possess an understanding of the social world. These might not seem different, but they are. We don't explain in order to have explanations, despite that one follows the other, both logically and temporally. Both the goal (i.e., possessing an explanation) and its pursuit (i.e., seeking an explanation) are borne of some underlying desire, which goes unaccounted for in this kind of paradigm.

Here, I want to propose that the nature of the desire that drives both the course and the content of all our attention, perception, and thought about the social world, which is responsible for all we come to know about it, has something to do with *psychological safety*. Note two things, though. One, "safety" is first a quality of experience, whether or not we use cognition, which abstracts and elaborates experience, to help us achieve it. Second, "safety" should not be associated with stuffed animals and hot cocoa. People can be made to feel safe by the darkest of experiences.

From this lens, all of our perceptual and cognitive discernments are in fact aimed at understanding, but not in a way that produces the most "accuracy," whatever that might mean in the social world; rather, in a way that produces the most wellbeing. Understanding in the way we do, whether action follows from it or not, fosters a desired state of being. When this is the case, the person-to-person variability of perceptions, conclusions, and attributions is suddenly accounted for. Different people derive comfort through different *qualities of being* and, therefore, come to "know" different things about the world around them. Somehow, we are drawn to those perceptions, thoughts, and explanations that help us experience that which we experience as security (whatever that might be).

Even if accuracy (or morality or logic) is what we feel we consciously follow as we develop our views of the social world—i.e., even if we aim at social understanding rooted in these ideals—we still must face the simplest, most piercing evidence that *experiential need* (i.e., comfort needs) trump our stated ideals: our outright inability (or at least formidable reluctance) to hold alternative views, once we possess them. It doesn't matter how or why we landed on the knowledge we did; it's our current grip that betrays its function. Whatever the force that led us to what we know, whatever our ability to identify that force accurately, each of us is motivated to preserve what we know for one reason: need of the *experiential* variety.

However, because the explaining, reasoning, and interpreting by which we generate them takes place in our minds, we tend to attribute our knowns to cognition, not to an experiential need for safety. We believe our explanations are meant to make us accurate (a criterion of value for thought), not comfortable (a criterion of value for being). The truth is, though, if we found ourselves gripping the side of a cliff, we would be doing so for the same reason we grip our knowns. What's more, if someone walked by and promised to pull us to safety if we gave the *real reason* we were hanging on for dear life, we certainly would not cry, "because this is the most accurate cliff!" We would be hanging onto the cliff because letting go threatens life as we know it, which is the same reason we grip our knowns so tightly: let go of either, and plummet.

But consider what would happen if you walked around tomorrow suggesting to your friends and co-workers that all they know is borne of need. You would hear claims like this one: "I don't know X because I need to; I know it because it's backed up by evidence!" We can all make reasons as to why we cling to X, Y, or Z, but the clinging itself, however we justify it with thought, is the signal of emotional need. Often times, those who most refute this idea have the direst need for their explanations. In a conversation about this with someone who I know to be exceedingly smart, she said, "it's not that I *need* to think what I do; it's that I'm right!" I hope the problem with this statement is self-evident, but just in case it isn't: what could certitude possibly be but need, only oriented to from a slightly different angle?

Thus, asking someone to simply believe in new things is not unlike asking them to breathe under water. Why? Because, though they probably wouldn't put it in these terms, you'd be asking them to divest themselves from their desire for their own safety.[1] Incidentally, this obvious but denied phenomenon has serious implications for how we clinicians might help people to change their minds. Most obviously, challenging thought with thought alone, or thought *primarily*, shows itself as a wildly fantastical starting point. Because something other than thought has moved people to their current conceptions (i.e., their current knowns), something other than thought must move them to new ones.

Striving Is Ubiquitous

The striving that pervades experience for each of us is the goal-oriented and discerning process embedded in our very attention, perception, and thought, which exists to increase comfort and reduce suffering by resulting in certain conscious understandings and not others—those that foster safety and not harm. Because the only requirement for this process is mere energy, it defines human being and life itself.

There is motivation in *everything*, and because it is a constant, we are apt to miss it most of the time, especially in modern life, which does not support nor reward *true* self-examination. In turn, we are often unaware of our very personal contributions to all we perceive, think, and know about the world; and at least in our default state, we are particularly unable to see that it is our psychological safety often dictating our perception, thought, and behavior, *full-stop*.

For example, from our narrow if personal perspectives, we don't perceive our boss as a tyrant for our own psychological survival but because *she is one*. We don't revere success or self-expression for our own psychological survival but because *these are the highest values*. We don't engage in conflict in every relationship for our own psychological survival but because we are *defending ourselves*. We don't want to crucify people who disagree with us for our own psychological survival but because they are *immoral, deserving of our wrath, or dim-witted*. We don't have the same exquisitely judgmental thoughts about our cousin every Thanksgiving for our own psychological survival but because *these thoughts are the product of our perfectly sound ethical system*.

The way we explain the goings-on of the social world do reflect something about the social world, but whether they reflect something valid, accurate, or otherwise is less important, less attainable, and more abstracted than what they reflect, most simply: a need so deep it defies words. This is despite that it rules our minds, unapologetically. It might well be the *real* tyrant. If we want to understand self, other, and world, as opposed to merely holding the understanding of each that we can bear, our minds must strive more freely. Somehow, they must become unbeholden.

Note

1 Even those whose knowns seem to create injury, not safety, might well feel safest amid the experience of harm. To be serious people, we have to consider such things (and consider why).

4

EXISTENTIAL STRUCTURE AND THE EXPERIENCE PARADOX

Despite seeming at times like one meant only to answer abstract questions about the cosmos, the project of knowing itself also provides us invaluable answers as to how we might be. First of all, it shows us that *we might be* in pursuit of knowledge, which has meant different things in different eras, and only happens to mean what it does in contemporary life (i.e., furious technological advancement). Unfortunately, once we have this pursuit under our belt, we go blind. We become unable to see either that the problem of being was ever a problem to begin with, or that the pursuit of knowledge is one of our answers to it. This is a destructive blind spot, though. If we do not see the whole course of seeking, possessing, and utilizing knowledge as a kind of solution to a greater question—i.e., how does one live?—we undervalue its foundationally personal function.

Whether true or false, valid or invalid, barbaric or refined, knowing what we do allows us to more seamlessly make our way through existence. You might feel compelled to object on the grounds that all knowledge is not the same—that rather than knowing any old thing, we must know certain things in order to benefit (maybe right things, accurate things, or ethical things). But it depends on what you mean by "benefit." Yes, the "wrong" kind of knowledge might move a person in an unethical, unsatisfying, or unproductive direction, but it moves them, nonetheless; and assuming the most fundamental task of existence is in determining "what to do," direction itself is arguably the most valuable effect of knowing. To understand why, we need only consider what experience would be like in its absence. Aimless drifting might be a worse fate than the worst of directions.

Knowing and Being

Imagine the horror of floating into space. Everyone has seen this image in movies, even if only for a second, before the hero is rescued or the villain drifts

DOI: 10.4324/9781003305286-7

off into oblivion. Why exactly is this image so petrifying? First, in such a predicament, we would be entirely at the mercy of our surroundings, wholly unable to impose direction. However, even assuming we couldn't direct ourselves at all, this would still not be the most psychologically disturbing element of this scenario.

What's far worse is that even if we could move in exactly the way we intended, even if we could do exactly what we wanted, *we still wouldn't know what to do.* In space, assuming we know nothing of its terrain, any given act is as viable as any other, which means our next move is, by definition, meaningless. Because we have no access to the lay of the land, whether we try to guide ourselves in this or that direction, or guide ourselves at all, makes no difference whatsoever—not because there aren't useful next moves but because we cannot know them. Despite the many horrors of this scenario, it would be our inability to assess the relative meaningfulness of any given act that would be most unsettling, since, psychologically, this characteristic would make us feel most alien to ourselves—most inhuman.

This shows us something about the necessity of knowing. It is strictly *the holding* of conclusions, rationales, and discernments that allows for action to be taken, for agency to be engaged. Only through *knowing* do concepts like viability and utility even come into existence. In this case, only in knowing a meteor shower is coming from direction X would it matter what we do—being adrift would suddenly give way to direction; arbitrariness would suddenly give way to order. So is the case in ordinary life. While knowledge is often conceptualized as a tool for *explaining* the world around us, to understand its most dire function is to understand what we would first lose without it: any idea as to *what we might do* in the world around us. Absent knowing, meaningful direction—but also the concept of meaning, period—disappears.

In these terms, all we know is not known firstly for its validity. Naturally, we tend to believe that we know things "because they are true" (and sure, some of our conscious knowns are true as measured by some agreed upon method). However, assuming knowledge is meant primarily to endow us with a clear sense of agency, as opposed to the clearest truths, we should engage ourselves in an odd thought experiment. Could we have developed any old knowledge, since any would have granted us agency? Or have we arrived at the knowledge we have because only this kind of agency, the kind we are acting out in this very second, would have sufficed? I don't know how this question could be honestly answered, but it starts one's mind down an interesting (and initially disturbing) path: "what if the essential purpose of all my dearest knowns—my convictions, opinions, and conclusions—was simply to prevent me from floating into oblivion?"

After all, regardless of the extent to which biological and societal factors seem to account for what people *actually do* (a science pursuit), there are always personal reasons to grapple, from within one's own consciousness, with the more personal version of this conundrum: "what might I do?" In fact, at least potentially, every passing moment has a legitimate claim to the question, doesn't it? And of all possible answers, not answering is probably the most threatening one as it fails to resolve the question. The key here is to see that the more we accumulate hard and fast knowledge about what the world *is*, what others *are*, and what we *are*, the less burdensome this question feels. In knowing so much, we've already "figured out" what we might do, and if we're honest, perhaps we've even figured out what others might do—even what others "should" do. Sure, we are in a state of dogma and ideological extremism, but these are small prices to pay to have neutralized the most dangerous—and most fundamental—question.

Consciousness is marked by a kind of earnest scrutiny of a subject that does not come with some immediately obvious point, destination, or answer: one's own being. We all must learn how to be; we are all forever learning how to be. Crucially, knowing—the drawing of one's own conclusions, the constructing of one's own givens—is at the core of this lesson, because only in knowing is existence supplied form. With knowing comes something to be done, a life to be lived. From this view, to the extent that it offers a compass, knowing *anything* has value. This is why, adrift in space, we might not see sure death if we suddenly noticed a meteor shower issuing forth from pitch blackness; instead, we might see our very life, by way of our very agency, returning to us. In knowing, paths emerge, which provide a course and establish parameters not just for being, but for being with consequence—for being in a way where *being might matter*. Then, these paths become us.

Behavioral Paths

One way our knowns keep us secure is by providing us a behavioral structure to be followed. Simply, in holding conclusions about self, other, and world, our behavior becomes more directed. Interestingly, the content of what we know matters very little to attaining this kind of direction. For the effect of a behavioral framework alone, the details of one's knowns need not look any particular way—they are arguably arbitrary, even irrelevant. When viewed from this angle, our consciously held knowledge begins to seem more precious to us for what it *does* than what it *is*, whatever it happens to be. Without knowledge there would be no direction, which means agency would fail to exist, which means being, existing itself, would be wholly meaningless. Thus, *any kind* of knowledge, any conception at which we arrive about the world, does something for us. Whether it is *inaccurate*, as we would say about the knowledge of cavemen; whether it is *offensive*, as we might say about the knowledge someone would have accumulated while growing up in 1830s Georgia; or, whether it is *unverifiable*, as a certain brand of knowledge is often characterized by omniscient atheists, the content of what we know—whatever that content is—contributes without fail to the structure by which we are.

We don't readily see this function of knowledge, but once seen, it changes the nature of the relationship we have with our own. When we know something, no matter how strongly we know it, we hold the assumption, even if only implicitly, that we know what we know for its content. It is very difficult, probably because it is unnatural, to see it otherwise from within subjectivity. For example, when we feel highly convicted about some thing or another, it is axiomatically understood—both by us and anyone within earshot—that what we are so deeply attached to, what we are so convicted about, is the *content* of the claim. But this need not be true. When the human need to structure experience is respected as absolutely vital, and the experience-structuring power of *knowing* is fully grasped, it becomes clear that we need not be nearly as attached as we think to the content of what we know. What we are attached to is the attachment itself, and we are attached to it for its capacity to press form into experience—to give our behavior targets, and our lives goals. Could what we know do for us anything more important than that? Crucially, this question is orthogonal to those about the validity of what we know. My point here is not that the content of our knowledge should be dismissed as purely arbitrary or meaningless or unverifiable; but rather, that despite the differences in what people claim to know, the most consequential effect of all such claims is identical: they help people to *be*.

Here is a concrete example. Imagine that tomorrow you were able to talk to a young man who has become radicalized into a worldview that warrants the silencing, censoring, and killing of people with whom he disagrees. First of all, he would not go near the concept of "disagreement." For him, his worldview is right and other worldviews are wrong. Now, what would he say if you asked him why he does what he does? Like all of us, he would lay out the conception of the world that fuels his behavior. He might identify his values, his understanding of morality, his view of what constitutes a good life.

What he would *certainly not do* is reference the dilemma I am describing here. That is, he would claim to hold the convictions he does for their *content*, not for the way he personally benefits from their *life-structuring effects*. In doing so, he might compare his ideology to another one, claiming the superiority of the former. But the notion that some "inferior ideology" is the alternative to one's own betrays a shallow understanding of existence, as well as a faint heart. In one's refusal to acknowledge the depths of human vulnerability, one lacks the boldness to see plainly the real alternative to extremism. The substitute for fanaticism is not another ideology but a life free of ideology, which is lightyears more threatening to any extremist than another "competing" ideology ever could be.

Why? Because letting go of ideology is to grip one's knowns more loosely. In turn, one must genuinely deal with their own being, including its mysteries, its lack of good answers—and because there is no better word for it—the *evil* constituted in *it*, and not in other beings (which is where the best [read: worst] ideologies always locate the menaces). The alternative to excessive attachment to preestablished ideas is self-examination; and when done right, it is meant to horrify.

There is nothing more terrifying than mining the depths of oneself with wide-open eyes; thus, there is nothing people are more loath to do. One way out of doing it is ideology. In rigidity, there are no questions: self, other, and world are all known quantities.

Although the treacherousness of one's own being is what rigid ideologies assuage, those assuaged by them are very unlikely to know it. As noted above, they see the content of the ideology as the draw, not the way that these ideas provide stability to their own being, and structure to their own existence. Thus, a hypothetical conversation with an extremist would *never* go like this, but his response below would approximate the truth.

ROB: "How are you so certain of these ideas? So certain of their superiority that killing innocent others who disagree is warranted?"

IDEOLOGICAL EXTREMIST: "Listen, I could lay out why this belief system adheres to all of my ideas about morality. But instead of doing that, let me just suspend the validity of everything of which I have convinced myself and talk purely about the function of my beliefs. If I gave up all I know, what would I do with myself? You see, my convictions might be valuable to me for a lot of theoretical and conceptual reasons that I can easily rattle off. More immediately, though, they keep me from facing the utter formlessness of my own individual existence. Because my ideological commitments are so fervent, they give me a sturdier foothold. I have believed my way to an existence with form. What's the alternative? Floating around this world with no sense of direction and every reason to look within myself? That sounds like an existence of chronic fear! No thanks!"

This example is not meant to malign extremists, despite that they hold bad ideas, by definition (after all, we all have extremism lurking, don't we?—careful, answering "no" might only reveal it). No, this example is meant to encourage the reader to see what one's knowns really do. Whether or not they hold any validity, whatever that might mean, or accurately describe the world, they always do something else. They help us rid ourselves of questions—those about ourselves, the world, and what we ought to do *in* the world. To the extent that we cannot see this function of knowing, we are wholly obstructed from genuine, reality-based respect for people, including ourselves. Even if they are different, other people's conclusions share a major function with ours: they provide direction within a realm—human existence—that comes with no map.

The Experience Paradox

All we have concluded, whether derived from empiricism or intuition, whether learned from a book or in a coffee shop down the street, whether widely agreed to or controversial, every drop of it represents the solution to the central human problem, one that is universal, can never be gotten around, and applies to every human being regardless of time and place, and era-driven axioms. What can both never be resolved and must be resolved, if we are to exist, if we are to have agency, *if we are to be with consequence,* is the fundamental paradox of human experience. It goes like this: as human beings, knowing what we ought to do is both an absolute requirement and an absolute impossibility. We cannot *really* know, not in some objective sense, yet we must know; what's more, we must know with a great deal of assuredness, lest our paths can never emerge, which is to say, lest we can never be.

From here, we begin to see something essential about "knowing," to which we are usually blinded. What we know, before attaching us to convictions, philosophies, or theories, gives us life. It gives us this very moment and every other moment. This moment—wherever we are, whatever we are planning, whether we feel miserable or joyous—was given to us by knowns at which we have arrived. Our very being, life itself, is moved by the conclusions we have deemed good enough to retain. From this angle, try convincing yourself that you are attached to what you know strictly for its content. We subjects are required to take things as objectively true, whatever this means, just so we can accord subjective experience with direction, purpose, and meaning.

The trouble is that once we have done so, we feel as if our knowns were just given to us, as if they are a product of "seeing reality." Maybe they are that. But they are also a product of seeking life itself—one's own. This is not to say that objectivity cannot be aimed at, or that certain conclusions aren't sturdier than others. It's to say that even what we claim to know "objectively," we know for the benefit of our own subjectivity. As we are dependent on it, regardless of its source or method, what could knowledge independent of the knower even mean? It only means something in abstraction. From within subjectivity, all one knows is one's own—and it is known for one's own benefit. It moves people to life, whatever that life is.

The Primacy of Paths Over Content

Regardless of how we come to know, only when we *know* do form, structure, and paths ensue. For example, only when the stockbroker *knows* that success is most important can relative viability enter into his experience, and can he seek Wall Street as opposed to the clergy. Owing to the order of things here, we wrongly take the form-inducing effects of what we know as something like a byproduct. In reality, existential form should be considered a catalyst for knowledge, not a consequence, though it is not thought of in this way, naturally. In day-to-day life, we feel attached mainly to the content of what we know (e.g., material wealth is essential) not to its organizing effect (e.g., learning about stocks, studying business, and moving to Wall Street). But we are shortsighted. We remain largely unaware that our real allegiance is to the direction itself, to the existential path that emerges from *knowing*. This is despite that we can see all around us, and since the beginning of time, not just that human life is a desperate search for paths but that almost any path will do. This can be said because, historically, almost any has.

How do seemingly sensible and reasonable people join cults? How do peaceful people become convinced that government-sponsored genocide is in their national interest? How do belief systems determined primarily by geographic coordinates license the killing of others born at rival coordinates? Furthermore, why do social crusades invariably violate what they allege to stand for in order to maintain what they stand for? For example, tyrannical violence at the hands of those on the *anti-fascist path* is still fascism; hatred of those less tolerant at the hands of those on the *tolerance path* is still intolerance; exclusion of those who are different at the hands of the *all-loving religious path* is still exclusion; and willful authoritarianism as a means of sustaining the *freedom path* is still tyranny. The list goes on. These contradictions, which have countless analogues in day-to-day living, reveal something extremely important about a human being's relationship with their knowledge. We are capable of abandoning the content of that in which we are allegedly invested in the very first moment its function—providing predictable structure to our lives—is jeopardized. At least arguably, the most valuable feature of the path provided by our conscious knowns is the fact that it grounds us, not the particulars of the ground.

Once moving along our path, however, we are forced to contend with a new kind of vulnerability, one that is systematically inaccessible to us. Knowing, which has provided our lives with shape, means we are no longer floating, but precisely by virtue of the structure it grants, our relationship with our own "knowns" acquires a quality of outright desperation. We need to know so we can *establish* existential structure (i.e., paths), but in order to *retain* that structure, we must keep knowing. From the outside, this often looks like simple conviction for the content of what one knows, but its purpose is to keep functional the experiential structure that content supplies. While our attachment to what we know is often far more important to us than the details of the knowledge itself, we are rarely afforded a chance to see it this way because the only way to keep the attachment in place (which engenders the structure and security we need) is to keep the content dear. And so, we do.

Rethinking Knowing

In seeing all of this, something important about human life reveals itself to us, something that is terribly difficult but that also holds infinite power to make us human beings terribly understanding of each other. All attempts at knowing are made by an inherently vulnerable knower, no matter how much certainty, superiority, or expertise he or she has come dressed in; and when knowing fends off floating, the most ferocious kind of knowing—that is, certitude—is always, in some part, a display of the most personal desperation. This line of thinking is not meant to criticize but to humanize people, to reveal something woven into the very fabric of reality, which is usually buried under our own certainty, assuredness, and "know-how," never to be seen—and for our own good. Once seen, it changes forever the taken-for-granted meaning of knowledge, our own and that of others.

When we acknowledge that in order to be with any purpose or point, we must first take things as so, our relationship with every single thing we have taken as such, which together form the parameters of our conscious knowns and resulting behavioral paths, falls into the category of necessity. Our explanations of the world are attempts to feel sturdy, and they are required by the very nature of human life itself, which demands that we know, yet provides no rulebook as to how we might. All our cognitively elaborated rules, protocols, and maps, which we allege yield the truest things, grow from uncertainty, anxiety, doubt. Before they give us capital T truth, they soothe capital F fear.

When knowledge is thought of in this way, what the knower knows is *most essentially* their means of perpetuating and structuring their own existence. One invests in what they know as a way of attaining direction; and once something is known, it continues to be known as a means of sustaining direction. Knowing is psychological lifeblood. Much like food and water, it keeps us going and moves us forward; when it is in short supply, we risk the whole health of our psyches. Whether anyone would *say* their knowledge is this critical to their very life, everyone defends their sturdiest knowledge, that which floats around their minds with total impunity, like it absolutely is—*because it is*.

Consider two political activists disagreeing and trying to persuade the other into a new perspective. Both would be encouraging the other to let go of what they currently know and embrace something else, but neither would budge, and both wouldn't budge on the same stated grounds (i.e., "the content of my knowledge is superior"). Considering what is being argued in this chapter, we should see that while each appears attached to their respective convictions, it is not the associated content they most need. That is, it isn't the content of which neither can let go. What *really* exists in the transitional space between one's current knowledge and new knowledge? To the extent that a person's knowledge is responsible for life as they know it, what else could exist in that space but death? This might sound dark and dramatic, but it isn't, not when one accepts that life as any person knows it, is for them, life itself. This is the only view of the other's cognition that will do if we want to orient to them with care, concern, and sympathy. Every other view, every other single view, falls short: each of them is *insufficiently merciful*.

Under this scheme, knowledge, which is contemporarily thought to represent the vehicle for human progress, morphs quite quickly into the vehicle for the individual knower's salvation. Simply, in holding conclusions, the experience paradox is much less visible, for after we have found structure, we don't feel like knowing is an impossible necessity. Instead, we feel simply that we know. However, the paradox is not overcome but represented in our knowing because the paradox itself mandates that we know, otherwise experience remains formless. We therefore never overcome the experience paradox, but especially not when it feels most like we have—when our experience is highly structured, predictable, and organized, thanks to all the things we know with certitude.

In fact, it's when experience has the most shape that we look around our respective paths with the sense that nothing else could be known; however, at that very same point, we are least in touch with the essential function of knowing, which is to overcome formlessness (and to give us a sense that there are no questions). This indispensable function of knowing, its organizing effect, is almost impossible to see, despite that it has made experience into something with discernable guideposts, which can now be travelled with know-how and sense. After experience has become structured, we are least attuned to what all our knowing *does for us*.

An interesting side-effect of this phenomenon is that the knowledge in which we most believe, we also cast off as most disconnected from us. In knowing something most assuredly, the knower feels by definition that what they know is independent of themselves, that what they know is so clearly indisputable that anyone would arrive at it. This phenomenon effectively absolves the knower from any responsibility for his or her deepest convictions. This should sound preposterous and unethical because it is both, but it is a very common and unthought about aspect of human experience. As the force with which we know increases, we take the content of what we know to be less and less debatable, which means less and less personal (or more universal). This is why someone can say "the filet is the best" and mean it from the very bottom of their heart, despite the obvious absurdity of saying anything other than, "the filet is my favorite" (unfortunately, this manner of mind causes problems for people that extend well outside the confines of their local steakhouse).

The Primary Function of Knowledge is A Human One

Knowing supplies us with a sense that existence is to be navigated in some designated way. We all need this. We could never do without it. This means that what people know—the knowledge they have derived—serves the kind of purpose that cannot be done justice with words. The primary function of knowledge is a human one. What we know allows us the means to exist with more and not less organization; with more and not fewer explanations of things that might defy explanation; with more and not less waywardness; with a more and not less justifiable existence; and above all else, *with less and not more pain*. For these ends, we will strive toward absolutely any kind of knowledge, *full stop*. And so, we do.

When we fail to see that whatever the knowledge we hold, and whatever the subjective experience in which it has resulted, it is ours, it is personal, and it was arrived at for the benefit of us, we miss out on the fountainhead of human understanding. We miss out on a picture of what us knowers really are. We are terribly vulnerable creatures, running around a realm in which we one day just found ourselves, armed to the teeth with the most ready-made but illusory fix: all our certainty and all our completely non-coincidental satisfaction with it.

From a perspective where knowledge is "just knowledge," and not "my knowledge," we will be afforded a behavioral path, but we will not be afforded a path to ourselves, which is what we most need. When we fail to see that all we hold in mind as "so" contributes to the way in which our very experience is structured, we are not permitted to ask why we have structured it in the way we have, as opposed to some other way. In being unable to reflect on our knowledge, its meaning, and its utility, we are also sentenced to taking it very seriously, so seriously that we will likely not revise it (even when we should). We believe we possess our knowns for their rightness, all the while failing to see their truer and less grand function: to keep us feeling like existence is a realm in which we—against all odds—know what we're doing. Our knowledge is only secondarily meant to help us know about the world; primarily, it is meant to keep us safe during the time we are in the world, even if our time is short.

Inevitably, knowing keeps us from seeing one of the many terrors of human existence, all of which collapse into the following category: a vulnerability so repellent that we can barely face it without having our knees buckle; one whose knees haven't has probably not faced it. When the knowns inhabiting each person's mind are thought of in this way, what necessarily results is a respect for people as unembellished as it is severe, for in a very real way that requires no dramatization whatsoever, all we take to be so—all of our knowing—is our lifeline to all we recognize as being. Because knowing what one knows is the bottom of *this life* as anyone knows it, we have been fooled when we see another's knowledge as something to be dismissed, repudiated, laughed at, or condemned. No matter what it is, there couldn't be anything more deserving of our respect. Casting others aside for being attached to different knowledge than we are, as the modern world teaches us to do in its impressive foolishness, will only corrode one's own soul as well as the soul of the other—the *latter* of which, when one finally destroys and rebuilds all their givens, shows itself as the very thing each of us is here to soothe.

In day-to-day life, we are attached to the knowns that give our lives structure, so much so that we fail to see how much human existence shares with floating into space, so much so that we fail to grip the true reach of experiential formlessness. It is precisely through our paths that we make life into something different than space—different than plain, dark, vast nothingness. And so, maybe it is different. But maybe it isn't. We know it once wasn't. In a time before our convictions, there was more wide-open expanse and less path.

Not only is *being* itself a permanent puzzle; knowing itself, before it is any other thing, is the way we put it together. And thus, certitude, whether in day-to-day life or in ideological movements, is a frantic attempt to keep the puzzle from falling apart. In fact, those most certain of exactly how the puzzle fits are often most convinced it could go to pieces in an instant, even if they won't admit it. Whatever the content of anyone's conscious mind or their worldly causes and activistic pursuits, everyone's *real cause* is existential structure. For this, there is simply no better strategy than knowing. And so, we know.

The Price of Protection

Thus, knowing is protective, but it also sets off another problem. In accumulating more and more structure, via the accumulation of more and more conscious knowns, there becomes much less to wonder about with respect to ourselves and everything else. Freedom from wonder is a strange kind of gift. It keeps at arms-length that which might *really be so* about existence, but it also keeps at arms-length that which might *really be so* about existence. As much as knowing sturdies, protects, and guides us, it also brings with it a proportionate imperceptibility. In knowing certain things, we forbid ourselves from knowing others.

5

THE CURRENT, THE OCEAN, AND ILLUSIONS OF FINITUDE

In drawing more and more conclusions, we grow our personal reservoir of taken-for-granted knowns. We hold in our conscious minds an ever-growing mass of information, the whole of which we reflexively take as "true." For this, there are consequences—and some of them are very functional. For example, having conclusions about self, other, and world is what supplies existence with structure, and lives with paths (as discussed last chapter). Additionally, it could even be argued that "concluding" is at the heart of the most useful human ability out there. Being alive is to be flooded, chronically so, with infinite stimuli and vast amounts of information; the ability to parse the signal from the noise in the face of over-whelming data, thereby holding in hand the *essence* of things, might even be a viable definition of wisdom—it's that important, that helpful.

There is no doubt that drawing conclusions and relating to them like they are true helps us live our lives. Yet this same process poses trouble. Landing sturdily on any given conclusion is to elevate in importance, even if accidentally and unknowingly, that on which we have landed. It cannot be any other way. This category of knowledge, *that which we currently hold as so*, becomes special to us. In blazing the trail of our mind processes—our attention, perception, thought, and interpretation—it impacts greatly the quality of our experience. In this chapter, I hope to lay out the mechanics and consequences of a tendency we all share: discovering more of what we already know.

Landing Somewhere—and Landing There Again and Again

What we can know has endless variations. We can know what is important, whether success, love, societal progress, or something else. We can know about other people—that our cousin is irresponsible or that our boss is understanding.

DOI: 10.4324/9781003305286-8

We can know things about ourselves—that we are short-tempered or light-hearted, or somehow both. Whatever we know, though, it cannot be known effect-free. Everything that is taken to be true impacts the future course of mind. Imagine someone who has come to a well-defined perspective: "the world is unfair." Whether they derived this "known" through experience or reason, whether it is valid or not, whether it makes their life better or not, once known, the knower will begin finding more and more unfairness. If they know with enough force that unfairness *is the case*, they might find it everywhere, even in every moment.

But what exactly *is* finding more of something after knowing it? At the very least, it must mean that one's attentional processes are different before and after "knowing," since what was not always "the case" is now chronically the case (i.e., it is chronically verifiable). A common explanation for such perceptual changes, and the one usually preferred by the perceiver, follows a kind of threshold proposition. It goes like this: when one's attunement to the nature, scope, and operations of some phenomenon (in this case, unfairness) reaches a certain level of sensitivity or perhaps expertise, one becomes increasingly adept at identifying it. The expert in identifying unfairness, for example, says that unfairness *really is* there, and he or she *really has* become better at finding it. Yet, we run into a problem here. If the products of our perception have taken a new form, so too have we. For a particular reason, though, this is hard for us to see. Because we have a natural and overwhelming faith in our ability to accurately perceive the world around us, to us, changing perceptions *could only mean* a changing external world. But this need not be true, whatsoever. All that is *really* required for shifting perception is a shift in one's internal world.

Now we can ask an even more radical question: could it be that our changing perception of the world has *not a thing* to do with the world around us? Could it be that finding more unfairness (or anything else), before it represents an improved understanding, represents, simply, a different understanding, one brought about by a different set of internal circumstances? As the newly perceiving perceiver, this is difficult to consider because we naturally characterize such changes as achievements, almost like they are software updates (think, "Perception 2.0"). We feel that our newfound perceptions, thoughts, and interpretations are simply more adherent to reality than they were before.

And why else would our perception be updated but in the name of reality? Accuracy, after all, is precisely what our minds aim at, right? Well, no, not necessarily. But this is what we believe, since we see ourselves as truth-seeking, reality-based, fact-driven persons. Are we not those things? Well, no, not necessarily, even though we often take ourselves to be, by default. And because we do, we believe instinctively that changing perceptions are the product of our minds having finally cleared the brush that was, until now, obstructing reality. In being so certain that these changes are a product of improving accuracy, we afford ourselves quite a blinding luxury. Why are we seeing anew? Because this way of seeing is *how the world really is!*—so we tell ourselves. But we'd do better to slow down and consider our necessarily personal contribution to such changes.

As changing perception goes, the perceiver is forever a part of the puzzle. If in February we saw unfairness twice, but in March we saw it 35 times, whatever the goings-on of the world around us, reason forces us to identify some change in ourselves, and not in—*or at least in addition to*—the environment, in order to account for such a shift. The onus would be ours, the perceiver's, to explain apparent updates in our sense of the world, however minor. One explanation is to say that we have become differently attuned. This is a simple description of the mechanics of our attention. We would be saying that it is now drawn differently than it used to be. But we are unlikely to say something so neutral. We are more likely to invoke values, which reveals something important. The moment we find ourselves to be *better at* perceiving something, simply for perceiving it more often than we previously did, we are about a half-step from saying what is really going on, whether we are aware of it, or not: that we take *ourselves to be better* for having perceived it.

This might not seem like an important distinction, but it is essential to understanding our attentional and perceptual processes. When appropriately understood, this characteristic of perception holds great power to account for what we find in the social world and what we don't, while making no stipulations as to what the social world contains. What's *actually out there* need not inform what we find, not even a little bit. Incidentally, to permit this to be so of one's own perception might well mark the beginning of interpersonal decency, fueled by a radical, at times dangerous, humility. This perspective demands skepticism about oneself and one's own mind, from which benevolence with the minds of others eventually follows. It is from this orientation that we relinquish the self in the name of the other; that we relinquish conviction in the name of openness; and more important than any of that, that we brush up against the divine. Now, let's see how exactly our vision might be a product of us before a product of anything we seem to see "out there."

The Perceiver in Perception

When we take something to be true, encountering *that thing* in the world is commonly thought of as confirmation or verification; related, "confirmation bias" is a commonly found phenomenon across the social sciences. However, this term is not quite right because it implies that what we know could still have been disconfirmed or unverified. In order to be serious people, we have to cut through such diplomacy. We have to admit that things we *really know* require no confirmation; thus, things that can still be confirmed are not things we *really* know. The experience of knowing—*really knowing*—needs no verification. When we truly take the world to operate in a certain way and then find it operating in that very way, we are unaffected. Our heartrates go unmoved. Such encounters hold zero confirming potential.

This is less obvious in the social world, so consider how it works in the natural world. If you were at a café and your coffee fell on the ground and spilled, what effect would it have on your understanding of gravity? Would it be "confirmed" or "verified?" No, this event could not possibly impact your understanding of the physical world at all. Your sense of gravity, nor your relationship with it, would be altered or changed. Why? Because this is what happens when you *actually* already know something. The moment one holds themselves to truthfulness, one sees that this is the real nature of knowing. It has the same nature in the social world, where happening upon things we already genuinely take to be "so" *also* fails to provide *any* incremental verification. We already knew how the world worked—in precisely *this here way* that we are once again observing.

However, while encounters with that which we already know cannot further prove how the world works (since we already knew it worked in this way), they are not altogether powerless to prove. Seeing the world "as it is" (i.e., as we take it to be), serves as internal proof that our perception works—*that we work*. In seeing something we already take to be true, what's proven to us (even if silently), is our own capacity to see reality. By this formula, finding more and more of what we already know would mean (to us) that we are becoming increasingly skilled; thus, as we find what we already know with more frequency, we take our perception (even if silently) to be getting "better and better."

But let's slow down. This seems like an odd formula. Why would it be someone's *skill* driving them to increasingly encounter some phenomenon in the world? It can't always be pinned on skill, can it? After all, we don't say that we are better at developing cancer after thirty years of smoking, despite that it becomes increasingly likely; nor do we say we are better at getting into car accidents after a stroke, even if we find ourselves in more of them. The reason we don't is because we don't find encounters with these experiences terribly valuable. We don't dub ourselves "better" at encountering more of that for which we are worse. In cases like this, we stick with a simple frequency description. Smokers are just more likely to develop cancer, not better at doing so; and after a stroke, we are more often in accidents, not better at causing them. Thus, any time we characterize our perception as getting "better and better," as we do in finding more of what we wholeheartedly believe to be so, we are not actually referencing relative skill, even if we think we are (which we do). Becoming "better" at finding something is, first and foremost, a reference to how happy one is to have found it.

The key here is to see that in knowing something, whatever it happens to be, a very strange thing happens in perfect silence: it becomes the knower's criterion for perceptual accuracy. What else could? Really give a few minutes of thought to that question (it's not so straightforward). In turn, finding it operating becomes evidence of one's own perceptual aptitude and adequacy; and now, one is invested in seeing it, motivated to see it, because seeing it has acquired personal value. Because finding it again and again has come to mean something like capacity, the knower will find it again and again, all the while experiencing themselves as increasingly discerning. But, again, they ought to slow down.

Changes like these, while they *could* reflect improving perceptual accuracy (if measured in some agreed upon way), need not reflect anything of the sort; and they certainly need not reflect changing *commitments* to accuracy. All they reflect, necessarily, is a shift in the criterion one is utilizing for "accurate." In other words, what's most required for external reality to read differently is a change with respect to what one takes as real, a change in the criteria one takes to *constitute reality*. Whatever the *actual* goings on of the world, and whatever that might *actually* mean, it's our reality criteria[1] that limit, determine, and parameterize what the world, to us, *really is* (i.e., really seems to be).

To Perceive is to Perceive Accurately (just ask the perceiver)

When was the last time you were driving in the middle of the day, and took time to thoroughly evaluate whether the sharp, upcoming bend in the road was *really there*? Given that you are still here reading this book, it's fair to assume it has never happened. This is how perception works. Things are just there, sharp turns in the road included. We see something, and we take it as so. We've just seen it, and so it just is.

By default, we and our perception trust each other implicitly, so-to-speak. As far as we are concerned, if we have perceived, we have perceived accurately. In fact, if anyone had their next coffee spiked with truth serum, they would readily admit that there is *no effective difference* between perceiving and perceiving accurately. These things operate as one and the same. This is the nature of perception, and assuming we use the same eyes for seeing people as for seeing sharp turns, things must not be so different in the social world.

But herein lies the problem, rarely to be conceived of as we live our lives: accuracy is a concept defined by weighing one thing against another. That is, it requires some criterion. So, we are left with a puzzling question: yes, we take our perception to be accurate—but *according to what criterion?* Whatever that criterion might be, our perception has matched it perfectly any time we have *not* stopped to question what our mind is returning to us, any time we have *not* stopped to argue with ourselves about what our perception is registering.

From this angle, changes in perception must mean that the criterion that grants our perception its axiomatic validity, the criteria against which our perceptions are weighed and to which they stand up without fail—whatever it is, wherever it comes from—must have *itself already changed*. That is, if one's perception is different, their criteria for *what reality is* must have already changed. If it had not, how could a new, novel, or improbable perception be deemed accurate? If it had not, how could we have a new perception and not argue with ourselves about it? How could we be *both* seeing anew and accepting our new perceptions as wholly valid if the criteria for "valid perception" had not already moved? If we are satisfied by a *new* and different perception, then the *new* process that yielded it has necessarily adhered to some *new* benchmark for "so-ness."

From this perspective, we accept perceptions, new ones or old ones, because they obey contemporaneous reality criteria. Our perceptual processes, if we accept their output as true and real, have been necessarily faithful to a very specific criterion: what one already takes as the world. This perspective would hold that the frequency with which we find something is, before anything else, an expression of how strongly we already take it to be so. And further reduced, if one wanted to make an extreme argument, one could claim that there is no distance, not a single molecule of daylight, between what one *knows* of the world and what one *finds* in the world. It's worth considering; it's also worth considering that one who denies being capable of such a thing is perhaps the most capable.

Concretely now, imagine someone who, in their conscious mind, thinks of reality as "dog eat dog," and people as "wholly self-serving." What would happen if, while walking down the street, this person saw what others would describe as an "apparently selfless act of kindness" between strangers? Could he see it? Could he see it sometimes and not others? You see my point. Expecting him to see it readily and clearly is expecting his perception to violate reality as he knows it; it is expecting his perception to disobey what he knows of the world around him. In this case, disobedience would entail perceiving apparent altruism, then thinking to himself, "I guess people *can* be good to one another just for the sake of goodness." As it turns out, all of us are very unlikely to transgress our reality criteria. In order to test this assertion, you might now be imagining all the times you *did in fact* see something that did not comport with your *then* working criteria for reality, which consequently caused you to revise your vision of the world. But not so fast—let me make two points about this.

First, if in sampling your own memory, you have found a genuine instance of this kind of revision, you have found it precisely for its status as *anomaly*. In fact, we wouldn't expect memory to store the opposite kinds of instances: all of the times one *failed to see something* that *would have* violated and thereby altered their then working view of reality (but didn't because it was missed). Such instances would not be bookmarked by mind because they constitute unremarkable, default experience. Thus, the fact that you cannot easily recall such instances means not that they don't exist but that they exist in such large numbers that your mind doesn't bother noting them. In other words, finding one example of a mismatch between *what you then knew* and *what you saw* is findable for the fact that minds note rarities, not regularities.

For the second point, though, back to my real argument above. This type of encounter—seeing something that contradicts one's currently held knowns—might be more than a rarity. It might not be a phenomenon at all. This view would hold that the event (e.g., seeing altruism on the street) did not cause a change in the cynic's reality criteria (e.g., "people can be selfless"); but instead, that the cynic's reality criteria had *already shifted*, causing the event—this particular interpretation of it—to have become *acquirable*.

This second formulation, the one I prefer, prohibits the world from simply painting itself onto our eyeballs as it never permits perception to be a descriptive enterprise. To the extent that *all we already know* is the criterion for accurate judgment, all the discernments we make and don't think twice about, and all the mental process that yield them, serve firstly as mechanisms of self-approval. Perception, then, would always be bent, it would always shepherded, yes, by that which one already takes to be so; but more accurately, by that which moves one's mind to strive how it strives (Chapter 3), causing one to take as so all they take as so.

Ironically then, for every claim that "knowing more" improves one's ability to perceive, discern, and understand reality, in the sense I am describing, it couldn't possibly do so. Knowing more would worsen these abilities. This is an essential but very simple point. Once we know, the course of *knowing more* is necessarily more governed because our perception is tied to something more defined. In turn, that which we can arrive at is systematically less and less free to vary. Simply, in knowing more, we see less. If we watch ourselves closely enough, we can even see this happening as our attention, perception, and cognition in the social world prove stale, predictable, and boring. In true honesty, we might even admit that we already know what we are likely to think regarding any future situation imaginable. Our *thinking* can become so formulaic and predetermined that it can prevent us from both seeing anew and thereby deriving new interpretations in the same way that wearing a blindfold might. Our consciously held knowns (i.e., reality criteria), wherever they came from, however they developed, seem to carve out stereotyped and constricted channels of attention, perception, and interpretation. Thanks to what we already know, the movements of our minds might be familiar and comfortable, but thanks to what we already know, the movements of our minds are restricted.

The Substance and Function of Reality Criteria

Reality criteria, the knowns we hold in mind and carry around with us, are made inevitably of concepts. Holding knowns in mind *is* holding concepts in mind. To glean knowledge, we must make moment-to-moment experience into something else. As an easy example, let's say we spend a lot of time with someone and come to find them very funny. Our experience will be conceptualized and funneled into a proposition. In this case, the 30 times Jeff made us laugh until we cried undergo an aggregation in our minds, taking the final, verbal form, "Jeff is hilarious." This statement, however, is not a reference to any of the 30, is it? The point here is to show that in conceptualizing, we make past experience portable; yet in doing so, it becomes a genuinely different thing. We could call it a representation, but what if it functioned more like a caricature? And what if at a certain point, it had to function like one? Then we would certainly hold knowns in mind that are quite far afield from the totality of experience that produced them.

Regardless of their realness and accuracy (however we would measure that), the concepts we hold in mind, as we are attached to their validity, have a real impact: from them, experience acquires purpose where there was not necessarily purpose before. This is an exquisitely important shift. Our symbols, our summaries of experience, are functional; and while they were constructed as a means of describing experience, once in hand (in mind), they do something more consequential than that. The concepts we hold in mind, which we take to reflect reality, serve to change our relationship with future experience.

When *what we know* is the criterion to which our perception naturally adheres (since adherence means our value), experience must become directed. It might not seem so to us, but in knowing, we task experience in a way it was not so tasked, previously. Subjective experience itself comes to serve as a special kind of barometer, one that measures both the validity of our reality criteria and, ever so silently, the value of ourselves. Obviously, we have a tremendous interest in how this barometer reads. Is what we know valid or not? Useful or not? Reasonable or not? These concerns need not be conscious to us, however, because our perception answers them in the affirmative, *chronically*, as it does what it does best: conform to our reality criteria, *chronically*.

Let's now look further into the reality criteria of the person mentioned above—and let's call him Harry (we will return to him over the next few chapters). Wherever it has grown from, his deepest held reality criterion, the deepest known proposition he can find in mind, is that "the world is unfair." Table 5.1 below outlines how his perception works to uphold both that which he already knows, and thereby his sense of his own value.

TABLE 5.1 Reality criteria and their effects

Phenomenon	In terms of Harry
1. Experience yields verbal summaries of experience, which take the form of concepts and are meant to describe experience.	By way of real experiences, Harry finds the world to be unfair; eventually, unfairness *means* experience and defines reality itself (i.e., for him, reality = unfairness)
2. Experience is filtered through these concepts thereafter, which means that the goings-on of the world are chronically "speaking to" or "commenting on" such concepts.	Harry could be anywhere at any time, and because this concept is so important to him, he (his mind) will inevitably ask in some fashion, no matter how subtle, "what does *this experience* mean for unfairness?" So long as he is experiencing the world, relative unfairness-fairness is always being indicated.

3. Because our own adequacy as perceivers hangs in the balance, we must take from experience that which sustains our view of ourselves as accurate and worthwhile, as someone who understands the world.	The contents of external reality that will confirm Harry's value as a skilled perceiver are those that are either genuinely unfair, hint at unfairness, or could somehow be perceived as unfair (even if it's a stretch).
4. Therefore, our perception and attention do what they can to earn us our own approval, which is to find what we already know.	Harry attends to and perceives (or mis-perceives) that which upholds experience *as unfairness* (and never fairness). His attention, perception, cognition, and interpretation are aimed at uncovering unfairness.
5. Step 1 repeats, as experience is navigated with no new information and nothing learned, therefore meaning what it has always meant (i.e., our reality criteria go untouched). In turn, we continue to experience in the way we have always experienced.	Harry continues to find the world unfair, confirming his view of reality and, less consciously, his own value. His reality criteria do not change because they are never challenged from within. In turn, they yield the same internal experiences (i.e., thoughts, feelings, interpretations etc.) they always have.

As this process plays out, we become more adept at "making something" of the world around us; but more accurately, we become more adept at making *the same things* of the world around us, again and again. As we accrue more and more conclusions, deductions, and givens, our own mental processes garner an increasingly defined and specific shape. Over time, perception and cognition take on an identifiable shape of their own, independent of the world to which they are applied. They then begin to function like pre-structured channels through which the details of the external world flow, as opposed to channels shaped by the details of the external world. At this point, understanding the world is still a process ubiquitously taking place, but something of a misnomer that needs to be properly characterized. Well-grooved perceptual and cognitive processes cannot be straightly aimed at an objective understanding of the world, even if we experience them as such. After all, the shape they have taken came to exist on the back of our own personal conclusions; and as such, they couldn't possibly serve to somehow "objectively apprehend" the world around us. Instead, they are enslaved by their *own* properties, their *own* shape.

The Ocean and The Current

Merely by concluding that certain things are true, we come to possess "reality criteria," to which our attentional, perceptual, and interpretive processes (unwittingly) adhere. Yet, the category, *what we already know*, has a hand in limiting not only what we can consciously take from the world around us (i.e., what we can conclude about a given situation or event); it also limits what we can experience in the world within us. Knowing what one consciously knows has significant impact on the quality of one's consciousness.

Here I want to introduce a concept that will be discussed throughout the remainder of the chapter and the rest of the book: the ocean of experience versus the current of experience. The *ocean of experience* is a phrase meant to capture the whole of the intrinsic world of being; that is, it refers to every possible subjective experience that could populate human beings, those for which we have names, those for which we don't, those for which we never will. On the other hand, *a current of experience* represents the idiosyncratic properties of a particular individual's routine, ordinary subjective life. Despite surrounding and even defining the perimeter of our current, the broader ocean is something with which we never come into conscious contact. This distinction sets apart the subjective experiences that routinely inhabit us (our current) from all the subjective experiences that exist (the ocean at large).

Thus, idiosyncratic, internal experience is carved out from something else. The way *we experience*, subjectively (i.e., the experiential current down which we personally travel), is fashioned from some the *whole universe* of subjective experiences (i.e., the whole ocean of human experience). The key here is to see that knowing what we do, has a hand in sending each of us down a very particular (and non-coincidental) experiential current.

Before showing how, I want to distinguish the behavioral paths (Chapter 4) from the experiential currents I am describing here. Experiential currents refer to the ebb and flow of one's ordinary subjective experience (i.e., what consciousness tends to be like for someone), whereas the behavioral paths discussed earlier refer to the manifest action one takes in the world. What they share is that conscious knowing precedes them. Both "what it's like" (experiential currents) and "what one does" (behavioral paths) rest on knowns so given that describing them as knowns "about reality" is inaccurate. To each person, such knowns *mean* reality itself (which is why I call them "reality criteria"). Let's now examine the current that flows from reality as Harry knows it.

Harry's Experiential Current

The deepest truth of the world that Harry can find in mind is that it is "unfair." As such, waking up to a wet newspaper, getting the flu, or being asked to work late induces a familiar quality of experience. He's not irate, but he's not pleased; he doesn't emotionally "spin out" but he doesn't calmly accept the situation either; and he rather expects that his future will contain similar, unavoidable irritants. He also experiences his broader life in this way. When he hears his cousin had a baby, a similar quality sets in as he immediately realizes that the world has never delivered him a loving spouse and better fortune. Moreover, were he to marry and have kids, he would still feel that life had sold him short, since some people with wives and kids have *better* wives and *better* kids; not to mention, some people make more money than he does at his crummy job, which allows them to spend more time at home with their family, who—recall—is superior to his. You see the picture. The recurrent conscious experiences that go along with these scenarios (e.g., bitterness, envy, reproach for self and other) only *seem* to be about the scenarios themselves. Fundamentally, they are about Harry and his conception of *what the world is:* as it is defined by raw deals, it could always be better, which means nothing at present could possibly be up to snuff.

Harry might not feel that he has mandated himself to certain modes of experience, but he has; Harry is on a ride—an experiential current—that takes its cues from his reality criteria (i.e., reality is unfairness). He might feel that he could attend to, perceive, and interpret a whole range of things from a given situation, only chooses not to because unfairness is what always presents itself—because unfairness is always what's there. But he is fatally wrong about that. When the world is defined by unfairness (his reality criteria), his experience is mandated to a certain set of qualities. In his day-to-day life, there exists but one experiential current that will adopt him as a passenger: the one that follows from what he consciously takes the world to be. His conscious knowns might well be considered a raft made to travel down one—and only one—experiential current: a wretched one, marked by alternating self-reproach, bitterness, and resentment, experiences that provide further substantiation to the same vision of reality that produced them (i.e., reality = unfairness).

Harry has no access to those experiential currents that follow from knowing the world as fair, or even partially fair and partially unfair. Such currents have closed themselves to him because they require knowns he does not possess. More bearable currents, about which he might vaguely fantasize, refuse him. They take aboard drastically different vessels. The idea I am offering here, appropriately understood, is rife with threat but also with opportunity—for Harry and the rest of us. It means opening oneself to the possibility that something outside of all one has ever experienced is *right there* to be experienced—and always has been.

Together, the knowns of our minds (i.e., our reality criteria) mean that we will take certain things and not others from the world around us, thereby truncating contact with the whole world within us. Though Harry cannot see it, there is a world in which he stops his fantastical longing for "a better family," and begins to experience gratitude and appreciation for his own. There is more subjectivity to find than merely the swaths each of us repeatedly visits. Somehow, every place we haven't found is also right there to be found, but finding it is impossible to the extent we continue knowing what we do. If this idea doesn't read on its face as acutely threatening, the reader might not understand it. There *is* more, but it exists beyond all of one's current conceptions of the meaning of *is*, beyond all currently operating reality criteria.

Current as Illusion, Ocean as Self

Just by being alive, we grow knowns. This phenomenon is so central to human existence that it might be strange to see it laid out so explicitly. In waking life, we give it about as much thought as we give breathing—it is so omnipresent as to be unnoticeable—but all of us are developing and prioritizing different knowns all the time, which are then brought to bear on future conscious experience. What we consciously know (i.e., our reality criteria) situates us in a particular experiential current, marked by recurrent and cyclical features, thereby limiting our access to the whole of experience, which is marked by much more. Depending on whose you observe, currents can seem relatively advantageous. Harry's, for example, is not helping him, which puts him in the position of wanting to escape it, while someone whose experiential current generates primarily satisfaction, internal peace, and gratitude would seem to have done away with the rest of the ocean to their benefit—almost as if they have conquered it.

However, the ocean is not something to be conquered. It just *is*, eternally so. Even if the currents down which we travel in day-to-day life give us a sense that there is nothing outside of them, that we are fully removed from the surrounding ocean, this could never be the case. We know this in a metaphorical sense insofar as our currents are so too made from ocean water. As such, they somehow simultaneously contain everything we wish they didn't, and everything we wish they did. No conscious state we wish were at bay could possibly be at bay; and every conscious state we wish were more available already is.

Whether our personal, experiential current and all its familiar characteristics feels useful or not, painful or not, pleasing or not, the deeper truth is that it *is not*. There is and only ever has been ocean. And each of us is the whole of it—all the time, in every situation, no matter what. The key, of course, is finding better contact with it: more contact with wholeness that defines human experience, but also more fluency with the various tensions, paradoxes, even the complete absurdities that animate it, so that one feels less pressure to make experience into anything other than what it is, and instead, freer to surrender to it, not with grievance but with both grace and aliveness. The ocean is the *real ride* and any individual's attempt to step away from it, to escape it, is the wrong tack, rooted in profound misunderstanding of what all people are, including oneself.

A wish that one could or should or might remain in one single current, or that one could spare themselves even one single element of the ocean is to reject one's own humanity for the illusion that perhaps one is not human after all. Such a wish is fraught with all the markings of conscious mind, bounded by what it *can* wish for, *can* hope for, *can* imagine—bounded by what it *can conceive*. Whether we can see it or not, admit it or not, a wish like this asks us to be something we can never be. No matter how things appear to mind, none of us is the current. Each of us has the whole ocean of experience within, and its depths are anything but limited, anything but determined, anything but restricted.

Whether comforting or not, there is no pruning the incomprehensible vastness of subjective experience contained within us, to which each of us is equally bound; thinking that we *should*, or that we *could*, or that we *have* is the fantasy of those who take human beings to be finite. We are not. There is always more.

No matter how out of reach certain waters might seem, there is always more. Every one of us is always infinitely more.

Note

1 Reality criteria, a term I will keep using, refers to the conscious propositions one holds about the world.

6

THE TENDERNESS OF SOUL AND THE DEVELOPMENT OF REALITY

Out Past the Artifice of Mind

With Chapters 2 through 5, I have tried to say a bit about that which motivates us to know what we do. Please let me begin this chapter by reviewing two major points.

A Brief Review

One's Own Input

First, one's own input, and thereby one's own desire, is required to know anything. This is easy to grasp when we know something like, "I'm hungry," but harder to see about the propositions that float around our minds as axiom. It is also difficult to consciously view our knowns as desirous because the deepest aspect of the process by which our knowns *become ours* is one we cannot think (recall the "unconceptualizable conceptualizing apparatus" from Chapter 2). Because we cannot think what moves our minds, even if we can think *about it*, our minds are disconnected, permanently in some sense, from that which drives them. Our minds can never contact that which is informulable yet propels it to formulate, that which is unconceptualizable yet moves it to conceptualize.

Despite that developing and holding conclusions feels driven by the simple seeking of truth, whatever that might mean, we rarely acknowledge in any conscious way that we *want* to know what we know. Were this on our radars all the time, the knowns we hold so tightly would suddenly have breathing room (and so might we). We would more often entertain the possibility that we know all we do for reasons other than those of pure validity, in turn relinquishing the "cognition as truth-finder" motif, at least to some degree. In seeing our role in

DOI: 10.4324/9781003305286-9

the knowns that populate our minds, much of what we formally considered *given to us* would suddenly appear *fashioned by us*.

One's Own Safety

The second major suggestion I have made is that people know what they do for reasons related to existential safety. In the absence of knowing (concluding), we would lack 1) conscious assumptions by which we can string together, attribute, and conceptualize the events of the world, even if all such activities are, at bottom, fueled by something unconceptualizable (Chapters 2 and 3); 2) any grounds from which we might act in the world, since agency only exists after discernment (Chapter 4); and 3) any semblance of stability with respect to personal subjectivity, since knowing about the world presses a recurrent form, whether helpful or otherwise, into internal experience (Chapter 5).

Toward Idiosyncratic Reality

To this point in the book, however, the complications and characteristics of knowing have been discussed in general terms. The text has not addressed anything related to the protective features of certain knowns over others. Sure, it is both true that we want our knowns and that they provide existential safety (as noted above), but what is more desirable and protective about the knowns at which we have arrived than those at which we have not? This is to ask of each individual person, "why *these* knowns?" and in the terms of this book, "why *these* criteria for reality?" For each of us, this very inquiry, the one in which we put genuine wonder to all we "know for certain" about the world, all we hold in mind that we consider "beyond dispute," is of essential importance to human life: only a radical openness to one's own innerworkings fosters the ability to genuinely see what one's mind is doing. What's more, even if we can never see completely into those operations that yield all of our axioms (which it seems we cannot), our interest in doing so is still essential because this practice heightens our awareness of an important reality: while what they return to us is often wrapped in a bow and labeled "undoubtedly the case," our minds are not truth telling machines—not naturally.

In this chapter, we will begin to look at the human processes that move individual persons to their individual reality criteria (i.e., the propositions they hold in mind about the world around them and take reflexively as given). In order to do so, we will continue to use Harry as an example, a man whose primary criterion for reality is "unfairness." Last chapter, we saw how this outlook keeps him ensnared in a painful experiential current, how the rather negative quality of his subjective experience is generated by his reality criteria (i.e., reality = unfairness). This chapter will delve into what generates reality criteria in the first place, both generally speaking and Harry's in particular.

Love is The Nucleus of Subjectivity

Without a firm understanding of what love is to human beings, it is impossible to understand human cognition or the reality criteria it finds. Unfortunately, developing such an understanding is not what you'd call one of the modern world's priorities, which means that clinicians and laypeople alike gravitate toward mechanistic and cause-and-effect oriented explanations of human life. This involves seeing what a person's mind is doing and attributing it to some other thing it is also seems to be doing. Such relationships are not necessarily untrue, but as they are plainly observable, they are too shallow. To grasp the deepest cause of all the output a person's mind generates—and not merely that output's proximal associations and corollaries—one must finally grasp the role of the ineffable, the unseeable and unthinkable. To start down this path, we must begin by discussing the importance of love in human experience.

Love and Morality (Love as Morality)

Essential to everything presented in this chapter is a simple idea: being loved indicates to a person that he or she is good enough to have what he or she most wants. The cynical might argue that people do not most want love, for each of us is *really* after things like money, success, and a well-viewed Instagram page. Maybe this is even true of contemporary people, whose very humanity hangs in the balance as technology makes so-called progress, but it isn't true for human beings at their core. Love is the most dire resource from the moment one is born into the world: without it, one goes unfed, unbathed, unprotected. Its absence means demise. This simple fact reveals that love, or care if you like, is what human beings are most wired to want since, fundamentally, it's what we most need[1] (regardless of how fervently we might disavow its importance later in life). In any case, whether we attribute our need for love to human tenderness (for the tenderhearted) or evolutionary necessity (for the hardheaded), as every human life goes, the importance of receiving love couldn't possibly be trumped, not by anything. It is the heart of existence; it is that valuable, that necessary.

In this light, receiving love means something more than just feeling safe, warm, or tenderly cared for. The relative love available to someone serves to alert them, on some primordial level, to their relative goodness: to human beings, securing love means being *good enough* to be given the most important thing, *valuable enough* to warrant the most valuable known resource. By this formula, a person's sense that they are *worthy of love* is wholly indistinguishable from their sense that they are *good*, since one defines the other. There is no deeper innate indicator of one's own goodness, not for us humans. And in this sense, human love must be the wellspring of all human morality: however quietly, the degree and quality of love that one is touched by, turns out to mean—*to the recipient*—their very goodness. On the deepest level, it means—*to them*—their own morality.

The extent to which a person has been permitted love is the barometer by which they measure their own goodness, whether they know so or not, whether they'd say so or not—and some certainly wouldn't. But this depiction is even too abstracted since this kind of "measurement" is not necessary: before the love that one receives is an important variable on the path to "assessing one's own goodness," it just simply *is* one's own goodness. The only assumption this perspective requires is one: that something within all of us, something rooted terribly deep, is aware that good things are given care, valued, and looked after rightly. Insofar as we seem to be a thing like that, we must be good.

Of course, some are only willing to say that the way they have been loved reflects how *others* have measured their goodness. But this is wrong and full of (likely needed) invulnerability. The ways one thinks and feels about oneself are testaments—always, in one way or another—to the ways one has been thought about and treated. There is a kind of person who exists to refute this, and we should be unambiguously kind to them, for one who claims to have gone wholly unimpacted by precious love relationships has often been most impacted by them.

The truth is that love relationships shape all of us. This isn't somehow true for children but not parents; the poor but not the rich; the troubled but not the well-adjusted; or Democrats but not Republicans. All human beings share this. Just watch people and it becomes very clear. In their way of being toward and with themselves, people show us something about *their* understanding of their own goodness, which was *always* first shown to them. Understanding the many complications of human life might rest on this simple truth—it's a truth that will never change, one to which we are all subject, one we all must heed.

Although there are many nongenuine ways to delude oneself into a sense of one's own goodness (e.g., money, celebrity, performative moral acts), genuinely taking oneself as fundamentally good—good at the base of one's being—comes from *nothing* in this world but being loved. When people with miserable love histories see this reality in the bright light of day, they are sometimes hurled, like a stone from a sling, into a new relationship with themselves, one in which their atrocious self-conceptions are handily discarded. People suddenly see that perhaps they've been seen incorrectly, and perhaps to their detriment. This can yield novel, kinder, fuller ideas as to who one really is in the span of two heartbeats. I think anyone who has ever seen this shift take place before their eyes has probably never seen anything more moving.

Subjectivity's Most Native Process: Intrinsic Investments in Experiences of Self

Because love is so important to people, because it means something so important as our very goodness, there is no instinct—no human process—more innate than one that attempts to save it when it is jeopardized. This is precisely what "the investing process," first raised in the Introduction, sets out to do. It is a process elemental to each person's subjectivity, which sets out explicitly to spare love by way of altering that which one *intrinsically is*. These most primordial investments, which each of us makes, are meant to *make us* into that which will sustain love. Notice here that cognition has no part in this formula—we people do not "think" ourselves into that which will sustain love; we become it. This process takes place in the intrinsic world, where mind isn't, not the world of cognition or cognitive representation: our investments yield an experiential outcome, not a mental elaboration.

To apprehend the investing process in action, let's return to Harry, a man terribly certain of the world's unfairness; and let's add to his story that he grew up in several different foster homes, wherein he was abused in every which way and rarely treated well. To grasp the purpose of the investing process, one need only grasp the simplest thing about Harry's childhood situation: experiencing it for what it *really was*—deficient, harmful, lacking in sufficient love—would have been less ideal than experiencing it in *some other way*. The investing process operates on behalf of this simple truth.

Non-Cognitive Awareness of the Standing of Love: The Mechanics of the Investing Process

In his situation, some part of Harry, a part he cannot trace with his mind, tracks *for him* the presence of love constituted in the environment around him. This isn't to say that his conscious mind doesn't also have ideas about the availability of love (e.g., "people don't care about me"); in fact, these thoughts and others like it certainly swirl about his mind. But the presence of love around him is surveyed and assessed most accurately not by his mind whatsoever, but by something truer, something I'd prefer to call soul. Souls monitor the presence, availability, and quality of love in the environment—and of great importance, they do so without error. Minds, for a variety of reasons, can mis-asses the true level of love a given scenario contains, but souls cannot. The read of the soul, a read unavailable to thought, is truthful, always.[2]

As the soul accurately makes its assessment of love, it does so with an exceedingly simple assumption: when people have problems with love, they have the biggest problems. To avoid this kind of problem, this same part of Harry, which *isn't cognition* and therefore cannot be traced or apprehended with cognition, makes an investment. This investment, which is not made of thought and therefore not known to the investor in the way things are normally known (i.e., via conscious mind), has one purpose: to keep love in good standing.

Importantly, even if one wanted them to, acts of conscious mind alone, like that of self-reassurance, cannot keep love in good standing. Imagine Harry trying to convince himself that "despite *these* experiences, love is still possible for me" or "my foster mom *really does* care, but her temper gets the best of her." First, such rationalizations, even if true, are not always available to children (or anyone for that matter). Second, and more to the point: words are just words. In such a severe situation, the products of cognition (e.g., new, self-imposed "perspectives") are powerless: sure, Harry can think new and better thoughts, but his experience nullifies them. Furthermore, all thought is fickle. All minds can change; moreover, they can be ambivalent, meandering, doubtful, and weak, and we can always disbelieve them, which means that a new "cognitive ethos" about his situation—even if Harry *really* believes it, and even if it might *really* help him—is always precarious. After a day or two of "positive thinking," he might wake up, lack the willpower to simply ignore the realities of his situation, and find himself convinced that love is never for him—and never will be.

Thus, if he is to keep faith in love—if he is to spare the standing it has with himself—Harry needs a vastly stronger tool than mere thought. He must not simply *think differently* about his situation; somehow, he must actually *experience a different situation*, one in which love warrants no criticism—only then will love be safe. The most obvious way of doing so would be to change his circumstances. That is, he could try to experience a different situation by generating a genuinely new situation.

This could involve persuading his foster mom to be less abusive; or maybe he could find a way to make his teachers less annoyed by his lagging reading skills; or perhaps he could change his interpersonal behavior, thereby making his classmates less alarmed by how unsocialized he seems, compared to the rest of the kids. However, as he is only a child at this point, his ability to effectively impact the external world in these ways is inherently limited. In fact, for no person at any point in life is there *always* an obvious path to relieving suffering through actively altering the conditions of the external world; and even when there is a path, there is no guarantee it will produce desired changes.

Thus, compared to our power to alter our environments, we always have more power to alter ourselves. This is especially true as we are first developing, a time of life in which our power over the external world is most lacking. And so, this is what we *all* unwittingly do. We alter not the world but *ourselves*.

Investments in "Experiences of Self"

Altering one's *experience of oneself* causes a situation, despite being no different, to register differently. This is the purpose and the outcome of our investments: *to ourselves become something different*. It is essential to *again* reiterate that this is not an intervention we make *with* or *into* cognition; it is an intervention *with* and *into* an aspect of human life more intrinsic than thought. It is an investment in the intrinsic world of being—an investment into the stuff that cannot be thought, into the way consciousness itself is experienced.

What we invest in are "particular experiences of self."[3] Of every subjective experience that constitutes the ocean of experience, we invest in one or few. This effectively changes who we are—or at least *how we are*—as it changes how we experience ourselves. Crucially, we invest in the experiences of self we do, entirely non-coincidentally. Ultimately, this process of investment into certain experiences of self (and not others), which is unmediated by mind, alters our situation in such a way that love finds itself—or we find it—in improved standing. To see how, let's return to Harry.

For Harry, the "experience of self" that promises to change his situation for the better is "self as undeserving." As this is only ever a mode of experience, never the stuff of proposition or thought, we might call it an experience of *undeserving-ness* in order to cast it more experientially. This is the region of the ocean in which Harry invests because in experiencing himself as undeserving—in making *Harry-ness* into *undeserving-ness*—his apparent suffering no longer indicates anything about the meaning of love or its availability in the world. Given this new way of experiencing himself (i.e., his post-investment way), love has not failed him: undeserving-ness warrants just the kind of love he is receiving (even if any outside observer would see it as deficient).

Although we are analyzing the manner of Harry's investment and the reasons for them, doing so fails entirely to help us approach its fruits. Like all of us, for Harry, the outcome of his investment is simply how he *experiences himself*. It is only a language-defying quality of consciousness. Remember that his investment was made from nothing abstracted nor conceptual; rather, his investment has made *consciousness itself* into something new, something that is only called "undeserving-ness" because we need words to talk about it. As subjectivity goes, the upshot of Harry's investment is simply *being Harry*; it's "*this-ness*" as Harry experiences it (a term I will continue to use, meaning subjectivity as it follows from one's investments: subjectivity as "this").

Harry's Investment: The Upshot

With this investment, nothing going on around Harry any longer qualifies as loveless or even notable with respect to love (which was the whole point). As far as he can see, everything is as it should be. What's more, to fully understand the inordinate power of the investing process, we must see that Harry isn't *exactly* deceiving himself that everything is as it should be. As his investment has produced for him something wholly experiential, its yield is no further captured by way of abstraction, thought, or conceptualization. His investment has produced an experience of *being undeserving*, which is precisely why he experiences no dissonance in a situation where he is treated poorly, badly, harshly. To the contrary, everything fits exceptionally well in such a situation. Given that in which he is invested in being, the goings-on of the external world (e.g., abuse, maltreatment) now fit like a glove.

As observers, we might say that Harry's investment did damage to him; after all, experiencing himself as undeserving couldn't possibly benefit him. However, from within his own subjectivity, despite having no conscious role in engendering it, Harry's newfound experience of self helps achieve the most important thing. Though the *experience(s) of self* in which he has invested might be harmful *to him*, it is protective *of love*, his vision of which goes unscathed and therefore remains a potential in the world: thanks to his investment, love should be no better nor more available than it is. This is the hallmark of human tenderness and the meaning of the investing process: it will invest in *any experience of self* as a means of protecting love.

Despite making life more tolerable, however, Harry's investment has also truncated his experience—as all investments do. Our investments mark a break with the ocean, in favor of a current. They make us into *less* than what we are. After investing, there are now things Harry can be (i.e., undeserving) and things he can't (i.e., deserving).

More on the Human Investing Process

The investing process can produce infinite outcomes and is by no means limited to people who are victimized within love relationships. Throughout life, everyone makes social reality into the one they *can stand* by making investments in certain experiences of self (especially those who deny it). Thus, while early investments are the most formative, the investing process is ubiquitous and chronic. For example, instead of confronting the pain caused by betrayal in important friendships, we can (unwittingly) invest in an experience of *self as invincible*, thereby subverting a collision with a difficult and painful characteristic of intimacy; instead of acknowledging that other people can make us no promises of success or easy advancement, we can (unknowingly) invest in an experience of *self as perfectly competent,* thereby protecting ourselves from contending with the ever-looming potential for failure; or, instead of seeing clearly the more mundane features of life and relationship, people can (behind their mind's back) invest in an experience of *self as perpetually vibrant, energetic, and enthusiastic.* In every case, the formula is the same. That which is intolerable about the true nature of human existence can be negated through a simple adjustment of one's internal experience—a simple investment in *what one is.* This is what it means to be invested in an experience—*and not in an idea*—of self.

Because the "experiences of self" produced by our investments are not made of thought, they are not known to us in words or held in language, even if they can be represented there: they are permanently of a different substance. The product of one's investments will only be found in being. We thus have a very different kind of relationship with them than with our self-attributed traits (e.g., I am strong, weak, smart, etc.), which reflect only our "ideas about ourselves." The upshot of our investments, those we make into particular regions of the intrinsic world, exists in conscious experience only. What's more, if we feel we have captured our intrinsic investments with thought, we have mistaken a *replica of this-ness* for *this-ness.* For example, Harry could say, "I experience myself as undeserving," but this-ness—the true yield of the investments he has made in the intrinsic world—cannot be propositionalized in thought or language. It can only be experienced.

Thus, the qualities that have come to define ordinary subjectivity as we know it (i.e., as we experience it), have come about through a ubiquitous process of investment, invisible to our minds. The next question is: what comes about from this-ness? What comes from the quality(es) of subjectivity in which we have become invested but which we can never think or say—even if we can think and talk *about* them? Reality as we consciously know it does.

The Development of Reality Criteria: The Experience of Self and Consciously Known Reality

With the investing process as backdrop, we can now discuss how consciously believed in propositions (i.e., reality criteria) develop in the first place. The experience of self in which a person has invested is marked by phenomenal qualities that come to feel most like them; moreover, it is marked by phenomenal qualities that are associated with the retention of love (but not necessarily consciously associated as such, since these qualities became valuable—and became self—in the absence of cognition). For this tender-most reason, they are the most desirable states of being. Whether the experience of self in which one has become invested makes them better or worse off, brings with them hardship, peace, joy or misery, looks self-aggrandizing or self-degrading, *it will still be sought*. But how do we seek these experiential states? How do we generate these phenomenal qualities when they are missing and preserve them when they are present? We do so via that which we have right at our (cognitive) fingertips in each passing moment: our minds.

The Makings of Harry's Reality Criterion ("The World is Unfairness")

At the time it took place, the experience of self in which Harry unwittingly invested ("self as underserving") allowed him to retain faith in love and protected him from the maltreatment taking place. However, as this investment was a genuine intervention into his own being by his own being (not a mere revision in his thought by his own thought), there are very real consequences. He didn't one day *think* he was undeserving; instead, he *became* undeserving. In this sense, he could be said to actually *be undeserving*, but not as reference to his inherent value or worth; rather, as a description of the experiential state he now knows as this-ness, the state in which he now simply finds himself.

From here, Harry's conscious criterion for reality (i.e., "reality is unfairness") can be better understood. The key to understanding reality criteria (i.e., the conscious propositions about reality that someone's mind returns to them), is understanding them as *consequential*. They are the conscious perspectives that follow from a particular experience of self. Harry's day-to-day attributions, rationales, and interpretations—all the conscious products of his mind—emerge from the ordinary experience of self that he knows in subjectivity (i.e., rather, that he *is* in subjectivity). Whether he has language for it ("self as undeserving" or "undeserving-ness") or not, his mind works on behalf of the experience of self in which he is invested (which in its true form, is *not* the stuff of language).

Harry's mind—all its attending, perceiving, weighing, interpreting, and concluding—is beholden to something deeper. It moves in the service of something else, something informulable, unsayable, and forever confined to the intrinsic world: the this-ness that, for him, *is* subjectivity. The key here is to see that the movement of Harry's mind, like the getaway driver at a bank robbery, operates as an *accessory* to the experience of self in which he is so invested (i.e., being undeserving). When this experience of self is absent, his mind aims to generate it; when it is present, his mind aims to further fortify it. Both outcomes are achieved by landing on certain conscious conclusions about the world. This is essential to understanding both what people's minds *really are* and the inherent problems of *being itself.*

In the following examples, just watch how Harry's mind works, while also considering that it is less moved by the events of the tangible world around him and more moved by the experience of undeserving-ness that defines the experiential world within him. Did he *really* do a good job at work? According to the output of his mind: no, the boss who praised him is a terrible judge of talent. Did the girl in the bar *really* like him? According to the output of his mind: no, she pitied him and didn't want to hurt his feelings. Is his landlord serious about giving him an extra two weeks to make rent? According to the output of his mind: no, his landlord is starting the eviction process as we speak. Here, we see that the experience of self in which Harry is invested leads him to arrive at associated (conscious) interpretations of the world. But that's not all. These very same interpretations reinforce the experience of self in which he is invested, the one that delivered him to these views in the first place. Now, let's see how.

The conclusions Harry has drawn about his boss, potential girlfriend, and landlord send him down not just an extraordinarily non-coincidental behavioral path (Chapter 4), but down an extraordinarily non-coincidental experiential current (Chapter 5). In knowing what he does of these situations, Harry becomes wary of his boss and upset with him, eventually being fired instead of promoted; he never asks out the girl he met at the bar because he "knows" she doesn't like him; and he willingly moves into a homeless shelter instead of taking his landlord up on the rent extension. Ever so non-coincidentally, he has not only interpreted each of these situations in a way that is beholden to his own sense of undeserving-ness; his interpretations have led to behavior that ensures his continued lack of prosperity. In turn, he only further entrenches his view of reality itself: that it is unfair (i.e., his primary reality criterion). And fair enough—the world in which he lives gives him nothing of value. He is right about that. What he is *deadly wrong* about is why. The world gives him nothing of value not because it is *entirely* unfair but because he cannot *at all* experience himself as deserving.

Experiences of Self and Reality Criteria: A Self-Perpetuating Pair

Thus, to the experience of self in which Harry is invested (i.e., undeserving-ness), his interpretation-finding, proposition-making apparatus is unwittingly beholden. Though only a familiar phenomenal state, the experience of self in which he is invested permits his attention and perception to find *only* certain things, which means he can interpret and know *only* certain things ("my boss is a bad judge of talent"), and not others ("I am a valuable employee"). The knowns he derives, in turn, engender a very particular and familiar experience of self (i.e., self as undeserving or a state of undeserving-ness).

This is to show that Harry's conscious knowns not only *emerge from* but *deliver him to* the experience of self in which he is invested. The way he experiences subjectivity, which defies conceptualization (i.e., the this-ness of being undeserving), and the propositions he consciously holds as "so" in his mind, which emerge from conceptualization (i.e., all of the propositions about the world that lead him to take it as unfair), are of one piece. They work together, keeping him embroiled in suffering.

The Bedrock of Human Psychology: Experiences of Self

The example of Harry is meant to show a more universal point about human life: the experience of self in which one has invested, which gives rise to this-ness (normal subjectivity) as one knows it, is *"the force for preference"* (Chapter 3) that drives one's mind to the conceptions it finds; it is the *"unconceptualizable coefficient"* (Chapter 2) that glues together and gives idiosyncratic shape to one's conceptualizing apparatus (e.g., one's attention, perception, interpretation), through which all of one's existing conceptualizations were inevitably run; it is the *"informulable thing"* (Chapter 2) that yields the formulations one holds about the social world.

Simply, the experience(s) of self in which one has invested is the ineffable apparatus by which one's cognition works, leading it down certain attentional, perceptual, interpretive paths, and ultimately to certain conscious understandings and not others (i.e., certain reality criteria and not others). For no person is attention just attention, perception just perception, or interpretation just interpretation; there is only attention, perception, and interpretation as they—activities—operate amid "this-ness" as one knows it (a quality of subjectivity that emerges secondary to the investments one has made in specific experiences of self).[4]

The Real Operating Assumptions of Mind are Inconceivable

In Chapter 2, we explored the meaning of assumption and searched cognition high and low for the one on which a person's "knowns" rest. But we found nothing. The trick to understanding conscious minds is to understand that nothing contained in them, no statable proposition or axiom, represents that individual's deepest assumption. The deepest assumption, the one that accounts for one's mind-housed behaviors—attention, perception, thought, and interpretation—and the knowns these processes generate, is one that is permanently inconceivable, since it is not the stuff of mind. It is the experience of self, which can be talked about but never said, to which all of one's mind-produced conceptualizations are indebted.

Sometimes I urge people to view that of which others are so sure as a product of nothing that can be said, not even by them, and to instead view the other's "knowns" as a road to the phenomenal experience of self they need. This practice sometimes shocks people into a relationship with empathic resonance, even those who lacked one previously. The stuff of other people's minds, which made no sense from the assumption that "people are rational," suddenly fits like nothing has. For example, despite making "no rational sense," Harry could certainly *be hurt* by his boss' praise, couldn't he? He would only need to construe it as empty, which is one of very few ways he can interpret it, given the experience of self from which his cognition works and at which his cognition aims (i.e., undeserving-ness). From this angle, it is plain to see why we people are often something other than perfectly rational: we people are something other than just minds. We are, so too, the unsayable qualities of experience that drive our minds, and after which our minds strive.

Intrinsic Change and Modern Psychology's Primary Delusion

I want to now emphasize the most important and overlooked point about knowing, one that follows from this chapter's discussion: thinking and knowing are not nearly the bedfellows we take them to be. Owing to the ubiquity of thought, we all believe to some degree or another, that we arrived at what we know *through thought*; that we can locate the origins of what we know *with thought*; and that knowing new and different things could be achieved *by way of thought*. We relate to all we hold in mind as if we came to it solely by way of our minds—as if it was our minds that invested in what we know. While this view is a bit arrogant insofar as it elevates cognitive stuff over *all* stuff, its biggest flaw is that it is evidently untrue. What we are permitted to know in our minds is constricted by deeper, experiential realities that are not themselves amenable to abstraction or conceptualization or representation or speech. The experience of self not that we *take as given* (a cognitive phenomenon) but that just simply *constitutes this-ness* (an experiential phenomenon), dictates where our attention, perception, and thought can and cannot bring us, thereby determining what we can and cannot "know" in our conscious minds.

Owing to our intrinsic investments, there is a mere current of things we can comfortably be, and then there is the entire rest of the ocean, which we cannot be; and what we can *really know*—the propositions we can consciously take as real—is wholly restricted by how we *must be*. As therapists, we want to grow a patient's reality criteria, thereby helping them consciously know the world as *more*. We want Harry to know that the world is not just unfair; it is also fair, among countless other things. But here is the therapeutic lynchpin: we must understand the force with which his experience of self (i.e., self as undeserving) subordinates his mind.

Knowing the world as more fair is impossible—a total non-starter—until Harry can *be more deserving*, since his currently operating experience of self (undeserving-ness) limits his consciously derivable knowns. If he could experience himself as more deserving, which would represent an expansion in *this-ness*, his mind would find new realities (e.g., he might stop finding "idiots for bosses" upon being thought of highly, not to mention "irrevocable fault" in everyone interested in befriending him). These conscious knowns are made necessary by mind processes that are enslaved: his conceptualizations of the world both grow from and generate the experience of self in which he is intrinsically invested—they obey.

In *being deserving*, Harry's mind would move differently. It would see new things, take new paths, draw different conclusions, and make different attributions. He would know new things, not because *the world* had changed but because *he* had. However, to do any of this—to see anew, think anew, and know anew—he would need to overhaul that which he is invested in being, that which he most knows himself to be, not in relation to self-attributed traits, self-conceptions, or any other form of cognition, but in relation to the intrinsic world of being itself.

Thus far, nothing has worked for Harry. Try and try as he might to *think himself into knowing* that he is deserving, these thoughts never seem to land. They are as empty as empty can be. This points at an important distinction: while he can *think* he is deserving, he just cannot seem to *know* it. There is therefore no problem in his *thought* that obstructs him from finding the proposition, "I am deserving;" rather, there is a problem in a domain eternally more intrinsic than thought, one wherein he cannot *be* deserving.

With this, we begin to see the strangest thing about learning, about knowing anew, the basic aim of all psychotherapy. If our goal is to help people *know new things*—the really important things that they do not currently know, despite wishing they did, despite obsessing about them, and even despite encountering them in their own minds but always in vain (e.g., for Harry: "I am deserving"), thinking could not possibly be the mechanism. That is, thinking, as a method of knowing, fails. But it doesn't *just* fail. It fails spectacularly—and it fails every time.

Whoever can see that talk about subjective experience is a mere rendering of the actual goings-on of experience itself, powerless to relay its constituent processes in their unvarnished totality—including how we *actually* see, how we *actually* think, how we *actually* understand, and therefore how we *actually* know—must also be brave enough to see the profound failure of conceptualization at large to capture *that which most is*. If we want to understand the subjective reality in which people *really* find themselves, we have fallen short by merely hearing *about it*. What's more, if we want to impact the subjective reality in which people *really* find themselves, we have fallen short if we are merely having dialogue *about it*, even if that dialogue is sanctioned by the sturdiest concepts, methods, and protocols 2022 has to offer.

In order to help another improve their mind, we have to become deeply acquainted with that which moves it: the experience of self in which they are invested, which is a quality of subjectivity informulable to mind, one I have represented in words as "this-ness." This target, the *real target* of psychotherapy, cannot even be thought (don't tell the cognitivists: they'll never believe you). From this perspective, what Harry needs most is to invest in "new experiences of himself," which only appears as a thing or concept because I need a phrase for it as I write this book. What this means and how it happens is forever more mysterious than we would wish (nonetheless, I will further lay it out in other chapters as a means of pointing the reader at something that can be gripped).

I want to admit here that my perspective casts modern, scientifically informed psychotherapy protocols in a rather trite light. Our procedures, treatments, and interventions, which we follow and which make us feel smart and expertly, are forever confined to the thought-produced construct world. The whole enterprise is a game whose players are collectively pretending that we are all "human thinkings." But this is ludicrous on its face. It's being that makes us, and it's being that makes our minds.

A Better Method of Knowing

It is in *being with* that each of us invests in our deepest held "known" (i.e., our experience of self), the one that lives only in experience, refuses to be conceived of or said, yet nonetheless determines the movement of our minds, including the conscious criteria for reality they find (i.e., every "known" we can say and think about the world). Therefore, it is only in *being with* that this deepest known could ever be altered, dissolved, or revised. From here, a better method of knowing begins to come into focus, then sharpens more and more, until it finally shows itself with so little ambiguity as to mesmerize whoever happens to see it. Some version of it first seized my attention on that day, almost 20 years ago, in downtown Manhattan.

What I saw, which changed me both abruptly and over time, both drastically and incrementally, and which I keep close to me in every moment as I talk with people about their lives is the very simplest thing. It goes like this. That which we *really, truly, and most know* in the deepest recesses of our being, is not made of thought, nor is it held in thought, nor do we know it because of thought. We know it because of love. Thus, if we are remotely serious about helping people to *really and truly* revise their deepest knowns, there could only be a single worthwhile method. And if it isn't something very much like love, it isn't worth very much at all.

Notes

1 The notion that wanting and needing are quite different is an illusion of comfort. If someone suddenly ran out of food, not only would a sandwich be best characterized as their strongest want and strongest need; they'd be totally unconcerned with such philosophical questions as to how that sandwich should be characterized. We can only not want what we need if we already have it. My claim above is that the superordinate human want is the care of the other.

2 This process can be thought about with a body analogue. For example, regardless of what you think of your relative warmth, some part of you not only monitors but regulates and intervenes into your true body temperature as needed. Think what you want about the weather—if it's 90 degrees, you will sweat. Similarly, people can think what they want about the relative love available, but a deeper part of them tracks it unerringly.

3 While these investments yield something wholly ineffable (i.e., a particular experience of self or a particular quality of consciousness), as opposed to something easily captured by an adjective, we must name such "experiences of self" for the purposes of this book.

4 It needs to be noted again that this-ness is genuinely informulable and unconceptualizable. It never meets mind. It is purely a subjective experience, which descriptors are deficient in capturing. It is simply a phenomenal state; adding the right language to it— or any language to it—moves one no closer to it (that said, for Harry, "this-ness" = "undeserving-ness").

PART III

Psychotherapy: Mechanisms and Meaning

7

WHAT PSYCHOTHERAPY ISN'T

The Limitations of Knowledge Transfer

A field named after the psyche—*the soul*—has lost its way. In our full-throttle pursuit to harvest it for more and more concepts, protocols, and facts, we have unknowingly disregarded experience itself. We have left it behind, thereby losing much facility with it. Students of modern psychology learn that intervening is intervening into thought—very particular, easily definable kinds (e.g., suicidal thoughts, negative automatic thoughts, thoughts distorted in one of a dozen ways, and more). As laid out in chapter one, our ailments and our techniques for treating them take the form of preexisting constructs, inherently divorced from patient experience. This formula pays very little heed to that which is *intrinsic* to the other's subjectivity and moves their cognition in the way it moves.

The purpose of this chapter is to demonstrate the shortcomings of our field's reflex to seize and intervene into that which is most manifest to us, thereby treating people as if they are very little else besides cognition. The world where people most exist, the intrinsic one, will not be conveyed in a patient's thought, nor will it be touched with the clinician's thought, even when rife with all the day's best information (i.e., the latest data, indisputable facts, and hot-of-the-presses interventions for "Disorder X"). Let's delve in by considering the following hypothetical exchange.

PATIENT: "All I've thought about this week is killing myself."

THOUGHT-FOCUSED CLINICIAN: "Can you identify 3 things that might help you to stop thinking that? I know you care very much about your family. How about just two more?!"

Here, the patient is thinking of suicide; therefore, the clinician encourages him to think of other thoughts, "protective thoughts," which might shield him from

DOI: 10.4324/9781003305286-11

his current thinking at the very least, and maybe alter it altogether. The logic behind this maneuver (i.e., replace bad thoughts with good ones) seems reasonable enough until we acknowledge its basic assumption: that the patient's disenchantment with existing might be remedied by all the right thoughts. From this view of psychotherapy, the patient above is well-served to conjure up all important "protective factors" that, once generated, will theoretically reduce the appeal of his current thought processes. As a show of reciprocity (or deference), the patient might even play ball. Minutes later, he might well be describing his appreciation for the fishing trips he takes with his old college roommate once a year, not to mention his beloved dog. However, the imposition of this stuff—ideation about positive things—is no antidote to the problem he is facing because thinking, whether suicidal or otherwise, is not the real problem. It's also worth noting that interventions like these, even when well-intended, are often driven by the clinician's mere conscientiousness, which is not always the right grounds for understanding.[1]

Yes, the patient's problem certainly has an arm in cognition, without which the clinician could not even mistake it as *one of cognition*; and yes, thought and language is one conduit by which we can get a handle on the problem. However, because it is the most manifest currency in therapy, arguably therapy's only currency from an underwhelming and objectivist standpoint, and because we estimate it to be capable of perfectly capturing experience, we simply overvalue both language and its most proximal cause (i.e., the thought that preceded it). What are we really assuming as we try to change thought with more thought? We seem to be assuming that negative thinking is the cause of negative thinking. But is it?

Some might say so, but this would result in a situation of infinite regress, wherein every bad thought can be pinned on another bad thought. Is that how humans work? Is destructive thought the source of destructive thought? If it is, what spurred each of us to our very first one? And was that one thought the starting point for all the ennui and dissatisfaction we have ever known? What's more, even if intervening into a person's problematic cognition seemed to change its course and quality, this would not serve as evidence that cognition either *started* the problem or *is* the problem. It would only mean that thought, on some superficial level, is tweakable. But such adjustments to cognition threaten to work like band-aids. Those of us who do clinical work probably most understand this—cognition is no weed to be picked or replaced. It has roots deeper and stronger than any oak tree.

What I am criticizing here is the clinical aim of rewiring deep-seated thinking patterns at the level of thinking. This approach is akin to giving someone a fish with no intention of teaching them how to fish. It's cheap; it makes us feel good; and it lacks long-term utility. Handing a patient a different way of thinking could not possibly be the same as inducing a change deeper than thought, one that causes their thought to be newly *and intrinsically* motivated to follow new paths.

The latter, of course, is much harder to do. As noted at the end of Part II, people are motivated to think differently only when they can *be differently*. The patient above needs to *be differently* so that his mind changes, only then will it stop delivering him to the darkest and most disturbing of places.

From this view, rather than actively directing his cognition elsewhere, we need to know what has gone so terribly wrong *in being* that suicide has become the destination of his thought. And under no circumstances can we be scared to say so: for him, suicide and thoughts about dying have become appealing. He is moved to them. His conscious conceptualization of the world is something like "wretched," and his conscious conceptualization of himself is inching closer and closer to "better off dead." Though the details are unclear, for this individual, being is a fate barely better than death, and slowly losing its edge. The thoughts and words by which he shows us this problem are only the most evident corollaries of the real problem—a problem of being.

Does Imposing New and Better Thought Change Thought?

The intervention above is one that asks the patient to suddenly consider information that, minutes ago, was not being considered (e.g., an impending fishing trip or his love of his dog). Let's think critically about the effect of attempts, whether by self or other, to rearrange conscious awareness in order to *prioritize* better information, which is one way to describe cognitive interventions (i.e., move *this* kind of thought to the top of your "useful conceptions of the world" hierarchy, and move *that* kind of thought to the bottom). Does being introduced to (and persuaded into using) more beneficial information really set someone on a different course? If it *really* and truly had the change-inducing effect we in the clinical world fool ourselves into believing it does, life would be different in several ways.

To name three, children would have been looking both ways before crossing the street since the beginning of time; nobody would have smoked cigarettes past the 1990s; and sunscreen would be as widely used as toothpaste. Unfortunately, it appears that bombarding people with "good information" lacks the power we wish it had as a behavior modifier. In some cases, our beloved facts even have quite the opposite effect. Have you ever heard of someone refusing an antibiotic for the fact that, yes, it might certainly help, but they aren't someone who needs help? I have. For this person, a former patient of mine, she needed to first reject a fact, then become sicker, and only then could the fact *mean*. Encountering new information of the factual variety has no guaranteed effect, especially not when it challenges important *experiences of self* (in my former patient's case, one that would be described in words as: "self as totally indestructible").

While this acknowledgment strips us of some of the authority derived from our knowledge base, it should also make us more thoughtful, more curious, and more confused about our work. After all, it appears that one of our most sacred assumptions, which follows from a view of every psychotherapy dyad as an expert interacting with a non-expert, might be flatly wrong: having new information might not be an antecedent to new behavior. It appears that, in fact, facts do not necessarily move people (and for some, they necessarily don't).

From this view, what is psychoeducation? Or cognitive restructuring? What is any tack the psychotherapist takes that is meant to remove, replace, or retool cognitive knowns? Is it a "Don't Smoke!" marketing campaign? It's not clear to me that it isn't. Why do we clinicians think new information operates differently within the walls of an office labeled "therapy" than it does in the real world? Unfortunately, as a field, we know what we know with such conviction that we have cut out our own eyes. Conveniently, we no longer see the most enduring and very possibly the most threatening feature of the human mind: that cognitive knowing holds infinite potential for emptiness. Our job is much easier if we see people as rationalists, devoted to "incorporating new knowledge and facts." Often times, though, facts are the nuisance, the inconvenient obstruction to be gotten around, ignored, or cast aside, in favor of what one *really knows* to be true.

Here is an example. I once had a patient who caught her husband having sex with his secretary three times in six months. Did this new information affect the trajectory of her life? No, not even a little; in fact, in her mind, she doubled down on her sense that she and her husband were made for each other. This is no criticism of my patient; it's just to show that minds need not follow reason, even when it seems most useful. Of course, everybody would not react the way my patient did, but some would—and nobody would be blinded to the facts before them. It's just that the facts don't always move the needle. As an experiment, walk for five city blocks, turn on any television, or visit any news site, and ask yourself: what proportion of the average person's motivational tank is filled up with "good, factual, and real information?" Whether we like the answer or not, it should make us think very differently the next time we feel deep faith that our logic and facts can change people. Let's now consider a logic-driven exchange.

PARANOID PATIENT: "The cashier at the grocery store hated me. What did I do to her? I had never even seen her before today!"

LOGIC-FOCUSED CLINICIAN: "Now, remember, you are only interpreting her feelings about you. You can't *really* know what she thought. She probably experienced you as an innocuous stranger and then just went on with her day."

There is no doubt that this clinician has more facility with reason than their paranoid patient. But why are they entangled in a disagreement about truth, fact, or rightness? The source of his paranoia isn't ill-logic—not to mention, perhaps the cashier didn't like him, and perhaps for a reason about which we know nothing. Was he hypervigilant and staring at her out of fear? If he's paranoid, maybe; and we weren't there. In effect, the clinician is attempting to teach the patient about probability (i.e., it is likely she didn't think twice about you because most of the time, most people don't think twice about other people in grocery stores); and beyond that, to teach him to rely on it (i.e., you should be guided by mathematical probabilities). Much of contemporary psychotherapy is built on the faulty idea that we can transfer a kind of "cognitive knowing" to other people, which they will incorporate *because it is true* (i.e., because we say it is), and utilize *because it is good for them* (i.e., because we say it is).

Let's consider another clinician-patient interaction. While everything the therapist says might be true as judged against the patient's behavior in the observable and external world, ask yourself how anything said could really catalyze change. Do statements like these actually help patients? And if they do, why?

PATIENT: "I've been unable to sleep ever since I got that B+ in Biology."
KNOWLEDGE TRANSFERRING THERAPIST: "The intensity of your achievement striving makes it very difficult to tolerate normal ups and downs in productivity and success."

While the therapist's statement might be accurate, I am asking you to consider whether and how it might help. Can the patient *do something* with the therapist's accuracy? Is accuracy an actionable quality? My general stance is that statements or interpretations like these, which convey valid information meant to function like facts (e.g., X is true), do not effect changes in the way we want. If they did, the patient might exit the therapy room in that very moment, armed with all the right information required for change (i.e., "Thanks, Doc. I'll just cut down on the achievement striving!").

But this isn't how it works. First, to assume the therapist is *actually providing* new information is a bit presumptuous. People are smart, resourceful, and can very often describe something of the problem. The patient above, for example, might already know he has a problem of excessive achievement striving. Yet, more to my overall point, even if this idea is new to him, there is no compelling reason to think it would simply prompt change. Our field faithfully believes that helping a patient to "know more about what's really going on" precedes change. In practice, though, most people have thought long and hard about their own difficulty. They often understand what relief might look like, theoretically speaking. But they find themselves unable *to be any differently* than they have always been. This is in fact the norm after one has met enough human beings. People are very perceptive about their own lives, their own personalities, and their own cognitive pitfalls, even without having been trained in the technologies of modern psychology (if you can believe it).

Think of it like this: if "all the right information" were the missing puzzle piece for people, we would think of 2022's smokers as the unlucky souls who just happened to miss every media campaign, every warning from schoolteachers, parents, and priests, and every unaccepting look from the social world that could have enlightened them about the health consequences of smoking. But it isn't that they *do not know* about the dangers of smoking. They definitely *do know*, just as a person in the throes of a depressive episode knows that sitting on the couch, thinking about what a disappointing person they are, and ignoring calls from loved ones is not the path to a better mood. Here is a related story.

I recently met an extremely high-achieving graduate student. Her presenting problem? She was procrastinating, destructively so. Her solution for this problem, prior to seeing me? Write out the complete list of steps required to finish a task, break it down into tasks small enough that her concentration and attention would not fail her, and work at it consistently each day during times she is prone to concentration. She even rewarded herself with TV and chocolates for completing sections along the way. Was she getting a PhD in Skinnerian psychology on the weekends? No, she was a person who basically knew what would serve her best. Twenty minutes into session one, we both laughed when I said, "that seems like a pretty good plan you have going," to which she responded, "Maybe so; it would be even better if I had any interest in doing it!"

Therapies "Informed by" Constructs

The erroneous idea that new information effects change is responsible for our field's perseverative interest in therapies that are "informed" by one construct or another. In such treatments, we see how our field's most basic and false premises have overtaken the hearts and minds of its practitioners and consumers alike. The solution to indoctrination is truth, and so what follows is my attempt to raise unconsidered and likely unflattering realities. Before we start, it is worth noting that it could be any construct doing the "informing" these days, but let's use "trauma-informed therapy" as an example since it has acquired special status as *an all but necessary* treatment for a certain type of person.

First, what exactly is trauma-informed therapy? Is it therapy conducted by people who know an awful lot about how trauma works? This doesn't sound so bad. But how exactly does this wealth of information about trauma manifest in the interaction with the patient? How does it result in healing? That is to ask, "how does it inform?" Here, I want to ask the reader to drop all assumptions *that* it informs and instead *really ask how it might*. I would suggest calling to mind the mental cavalry with no loyalties to givens, no interest in accommodating norms for the sake of it, and total freedom from the need to be an upright and responsible clinician committed to the day's sturdiest advances. Good, now we can think about this issue unbounded by rules—with more honesty and less fear.

Yes, trauma-informed therapy is a therapeutic encounter informed by all kinds of information and facts about trauma. This can be said because in the contemporary psychology world, trauma, like every construct, is defined by nothing if not the facts by which it is constituted, those that research has revealed. This is why some in our field would be aghast at the prospect of sending a traumatized person to a clinician unarmed with all of the *agreed upon facts* about trauma. They see our DSM constructs (e.g., Post Traumatic Stress Disorder [PTSD] vs. Generalized Anxiety Disorder [GAD]) as constituted by very specific and distinct properties, which are distinguishable by observation and best treated with corresponding methods (trauma-informed therapy vs. Cognitive-Behavioral Therapy [CBT] for anxiety). This view holds that something like "adjustment disorder with anxiety" is *quite a different animal* than "adjustment disorder with mixed anxiety and depressed mood."[2]

In our field's view, trauma is certainly a thing in itself, defined by the facts and correlates that make it what it is; and treatment for trauma is a second thing in itself, defined by those methods that diminish the presentation of the first thing. Both constructs (trauma) and our construct-influencers (trauma-informed treatment) are things that we know about. They are things, out there in the world, comprised by facts and about which more and more facts can be corralled. Modern psychology rests on unearthing constructs, then knowing more and more about them. Given all of this, we must believe that the value of having an expert in the therapy room rests on the whole universe of things he or she *knows about*. After all, knowing *about*—knowing *a lot about*—defines expertise; and what are "trauma-informed therapists" but experts *about* trauma? Theoretically, trauma experts have more cognitive access to information about trauma than others do.

This information might include facts about who becomes traumatized and why; which events make trauma symptoms worse; and when, how, and why hypervigilance floods the perceptual processes of trauma survivors. Now, instead of just assuming that facts about trauma are actionable, let's try to figure out *exactly* how they might be. Is this kind of expert meant to be a master-psycho-educator? And does the masterful psychoeducation of a patient constitute useful therapy? Some might believe so, but recall that psychotherapy takes place *in being*, not in *about being*, the latter of which is the domain from which all "psychoeducative" content hails. Because critiques like the one I am making are assaultive to our modern, scientistic sensibilities, they cannot be taken seriously; in turn, we cannot see something that is plainly evident: the most valuable thing for a clinician to "know" as it relates to trauma is how to *be with this* traumatized person in *this moment*. Despite that most of our field assumes there is one, what is the *axiomatic reason* to think that facts about trauma (i.e., cognitive knowing) would foster this latter kind of knowing?

That is, why do we think good facts translate ever-so-perfectly into useful here-and-now encounters? This is not to say that certified "trauma therapists" aren't wonderful and extraordinarily good for people. I know many who are, and one with whom I regularly consult. But it isn't her "knowledge about" that makes her so good for people, not primarily. We should be braver about admitting such things (even if it's a thorn in the side of our expertise—and it is).

Facts and Experience: An Oxymoronic Union

What is a psychological fact in moment-to-moment experience? Of trauma, one *fact* is that people who have endured something terrible tend to experience hypervigilance and hyperarousal more readily, which means a much lower threshold for things like panic, worry, agitation, and paranoia. How did this information, which is all true, become true? These phenomena have become "fact" by way of a systematic process of observation, which allows us to say that certain things go together. Our observations are pressed into forms (e.g., variables), and said to co-occur. In this case, noxious events (variable one) seem to occur alongside increasing bodily and psychological reactivity (variable two). But this is where things get a little harder to think about: do such relationships exist in subjective experience? In the world of non-abstracted being, not only do facts not have special status; it's also unclear to what they refer.

Subjectivity itself, not subjectivity as conceptualized, is this moment, whereas facts are abstracted from multiple moments. In *this moment*, we can surely think about facts and refer to them in our thoughts and words, but this moment itself is defined singularly by the all-encompassing, conscious, phenomenal quality that presently grips us; and importantly, while this quality, whatever it is, might be brought about by myriad things, it is experienced as one thing. It is a non-reducible whole. Regardless of whatever caused it, however long it will persist, or what gave rise to it, *this* is the only state that *is*. As experience goes, you and I are right now populated, simply, by *this-ness*.

While psychological facts might be represented by mind, we should be less sure that they exist in consciousness itself. Despite our capacity to construct them with incredible precision and accuracy, has anyone ever *experienced* a fact? Facts are true insofar as they show valid and actual relationships between phenomena, but the moment we ask what a fact *really is* in terms of subjective experience, problems emerge. Here is an analogy. While it is true that consciousness exists over time, say over a period of an hour, "an hour" has no representation in consciousness. Nobody has ever experienced "an hour," despite having experienced every moment by which it was constituted.

Facts, since they are only concepts, even if surefire ones, are not the stuff of the being realm, which can only be defined as that in subjectivity, which *homogenously* and *currently is*. To see this concretely, ask yourself if a trauma survivor can ever experience this fact: "since experiencing this or that brutality, my nervous system has changed in such a way that I am now much more sensitive to things that I have not been sensitive to in the past." This might be deadly true; in this moment, however, it exists strictly as a conception, as an inhabitant of elaborated thought. There is no experiential correlate for explanations, truths, or facts, which have been assembled by the mind, no matter how "true," when experience is simply *this*, and no more.

Facts require *more time* than the present moment as they develop over whatever timespan a fact-finding mission is carried out; they require *a methodology*, which itself has no representation in conscious experience but through which consciousness is strung together so that meaningful relationships between phenomena can be solidified; and they require *more people* than just the subject of subjective experience, and therefore might be considered the aggregate of several subjective experiences (i.e., N=30). Psychological facts are not derived from consciousness as experienced but from consciousness as represented. Arguably then, they are not quantities to be experienced.

A Hook for Facts? Or an Illusion?

Imagine meeting a new patient, someone who has endured multiple traumatic experiences beginning in childhood. She tells you that on the way to your office she had a frightening encounter on the bus, which prompted a ruminative process. Now, she can barely think straight and is very worried that someone is after her. There is nothing wrong with assuming, "the episode on the bus was somehow reminiscent of old relationships or experiences, which has put her in a fearful state and thrown a wrench into her cognition." This might be true, and it might be considered a kind of fact, meaning that this explanation, from start to finish, might well capture the course of events that has given way to consciousness as she is now experiencing it (this-ness). However, despite its effectiveness in *accounting for* the quality of her conscious experience, this explanation does not *itself* exist in her conscious experience. What exists there is only that which is *now* gripping her—*and nothing else*—which is nothing like a fact.

Being guided by such abstractions, then, is to be guided by something other than *what is*. Our obsession with facts has caused us in psychology to forget the very thing our facts allegedly hold promise to improve: the conscious experience of human beings. This could cause us clinicians to grapple with a real problem related to our attention; it could force us to consider the extent to which we value *what is* (i.e., here-and-now conscious experience), as compared to what *we think is* (i.e., everything else). If we have found a hook within the encounter to which we can seamlessly fasten our facts, we have one foot, necessarily and by definition, outside of the encounter.

We say our facts inform the encounter, but if nothing about the encounter itself informed our facts, then why do we ascribe these facts so much utility? In other words, how did these facts become so important? Why not sit a trauma survivor down across from a historian, chock-full of facts about the civil war? This might seem like a strange (and admittedly polemical) proposition until we consider that *his facts* and *facts about trauma* were equally generated by that patient's idiosyncratic experience. That is, they weren't—not at all. If we have invoked interventions that we characterize as "informed by facts," we have necessarily left the world of experience for a world of abstraction, which reveals something important. That which is a-priori and methodology produced—*that which does the informing* in trauma-informed interactions—has no origins in the interaction itself. From this perspective, it seems that entire interactions are not "informed" by expert-level cognitive knowledge (e.g., about Construct X) but dictated by it. This has a less appealing ring to it, no?

What's more, if the whole therapy is slowly moving toward the patient's new understanding of that which the therapist already understands (e.g., what trauma is and how to improve it), then relative progress, which is usually defined by the patient's improved well-being, becomes synonymous with the speed and fury with which the practitioner can transfer new knowledge. Viewed from his angle, therapies informed by this or that threaten to reduce to a kind of sale. Are such treatments responding to the patient's experience or to a-priori facts, which were produced by many people (e.g., N=150) who are not the patient? Is it even possible to respond to both?

Time to Tell the Truth: The Expression of Values, Not the Delivery of Facts

The way patients are impacted in here-and-now consciousness has only so much to do with the content or accuracy of the verbal information we supply, or the underlying operations through which that information was produced. Even when we are conveying facts, we are conveying ourselves, a way of being, a presence, a quality of consciousness, to which the patient's quality of consciousness, as it currently stands, responds. When one thinks about what facts really are, it makes sense that they would not move the living. They are, after all, black and white, objective, and lifeless.

Not only do facts not exist in moment-to-moment experience (as laid out above); they aren't supposed to. The property of a fact that makes it valuable is that it does away with subjectivity; a fact is meant to usher in pure objectivity. Despite that facts are meant to cancel all the "error and noise" *of individual experience*, once we in psychology have a hold of them, we proceed to proudly apply them to this very same domain. This means something quite obvious that cannot be talked about within a field so possessed by science. If a patient's subjective experience seems to be improving in response to being delivered facts (e.g., after being conveyed psychoeducation, information about disorders, information about treatments), or while being treated with methods based on facts (e.g., any empirically supported treatment protocol), we—in characteristic fashion—should be thinking harder. Something else is most certainly going on.

Let's imagine a clinical moment in which a patient wants to know what qualifies them as "having PTSD." It's worth noting that people don't by their nature want to medicalize their own experience, but our field's reverence for robotics—symptom lists, checkboxes, and categories—has made its way into the general public's consciousness, causing the deferent to happily reduce their idiosyncratic experience to labels. That aside, in response to this patient's question, we could provide an empirically supported, developmental theory about the origins and effects of maltreatment while matching what we know of the patient's history to the model. We could also recite the symptoms from the DSM for which we believe the patient "meets criteria." Either approach would in fact be a valid response insofar as both are rooted in what we could defensibly call "facts." However, instead of rifling through our warehouse of expert knowledge, let's instead aim to care, precisely and singularly, about the *meaning* of a question like this. What is *actually happening* in the room when a traumatized patient asks a clinician for some knowledge and guidance about their problems?

First of all, the relative utility of our response to a question like this has much more to do with our ability to *be in the right way* than with *being right*; more to do with *how we are* and less to do with *what we say*. A trauma victim's dilemma is real, unabstracted. It is always operating. It exists in real time with real humans. This includes us, the clinician, an authority who people have no reason to trust, except for buying into the rules of the mental health game and doing so on faith. But these rules (i.e., "clinicians are benevolent"), much like patient diagnoses, are abstractions. The here-and-now reality makes plenty of room for our potential for harm. On some level, the patient knows this about us. If they don't see in us any potential for harm, they are naïve; and if we don't, we are at least naïve, likely dishonest, and certainly strangers to the whole of ourselves.

A patient asking about constructs (e.g., PTSD) and their contents (e.g., hypervigilance), is also asking to be shown something—perhaps not consciously or even intentionally, but even so, her eyes are on us. Maybe she wants to see how we deal with power; maybe she wants to see if we can be trusted; and maybe we picked up on these motivations because of the way she betrayed, in the course of one millisecond, an expression that said, "people are bad to me." And maybe, somehow, we know this is true, but not as true as she thinks; or maybe somehow, we see that she's understating the true degree of injury she feels. None of this was said, but all of it complicates the stated question, "what's my diagnosis?" As a clinician in a situation like this, calling on and offering the cognitive knowledge of the construct world (e.g., theoretical models of trauma, DSM lists) is to say something that is perfectly true, but to be something that is perfectly hollow.

For Maya: A Brief Case Example

Imagine a girl who was often kept home from school throughout childhood solely because her mother was lonely and could not tolerate the separation. To keep the patient attached, her mother made a practice of lying to her about her health, at times made her sick intentionally, and always kept her totally uninformed and confused about the state of her own health. As a child, she had no idea what was true and what wasn't about her health; she only knew that her mom was always sufficiently concerned as to keep her home from school. Now imagine she comes to see you as an adult. In DSM lingo, she has presented for "chronic PTSD"—a fair enough diagnosis. But the problem she really wants your help with is more basic, more human, and more touching, if we only let ourselves be touched by it. The problem? If we drop our Pollyannaish tendencies, which we must, we immediately see that Maya has every reason in the world to give up on people completely, and though she doesn't *really want to*, she also *really does*; and maybe she is so compelling that part of us thinks she should!

She is engaged in an intrapsychic war about the basic state of humanity. Are people harmful? Is her mom evil? Is *she* evil for thinking her mom might be? Can she find a good life amongst humans, who appear to her both as saviors (i.e., Mom as idealized nurse) and pathetic creatures who direct their own pain at their daughters in the form of pure malevolence (i.e., Mom as malignant controller)? These are not technical questions about sterile constructs, are they? These are questions about love and hatred, good and evil, divinity and wickedness (concepts curiously missing from the DSM); and being soulful, alive, and awake—and not soulless, deadened, or asleep—is to identify them as such. Now that we know she has a love problem, primarily, what does it mean when Maya asks us about something so profanely technical as classification (e.g., "what criteria do I meet?").

If we are not careful with this question, we will be quickly pulled out of the tender world of being and into the sterile world of "fact." In asking her question, we see that she is dying to hear what we think. Her consciousness is receptive, earnest, and eagerly awaiting our facts. But she doesn't want facts for the sake of facts, and her earnestness tells us so. Facts are impartial. She is not. She is extremely engaged, and we can feel the intensity of her attention registering in our consciousness. She is showing us how important this information is. Why, though? Because, strangely enough, kindly outlining a list of sterile DSM symptoms, however technical and robotic, might not seem so to her. It might be precisely what she needs. Remember that a lack of straight answers about her health—about herself—is what first harmed her. A lack of straight answers compromised her ability to have any practice with self-possession, power, or agency. She is a person whose relationship with close others has been defined, more than anything, by deceit. And so, what does she need from us? Facts? No! We need to *be someone* with zero reluctance and zero qualms about being entirely transparent. This is the right way to *know her*, regardless of what else we might also *know about trauma*.

Supposing we did list five symptoms that fit her presentation, it is important to remember that the "empirical accuracy" of our response is not what makes it the best response; it's solely the unsaid meaning, which is transferred to the patient in experience, not words, and touches them in being, not cognition. After all, as far as her cognition is concerned, we just listed off some symptoms. But this is *not at all* what happened. We showed her something of which words were merely a necessary component. In doing so, we might have provided her the tiniest, and very possibly the first piece of evidence that faith in humanity, particularly authority, could be a worthwhile stance. At least in our office, maybe she could *be someone* of sufficient value to be told the whole truth. The therapeutic action was to say the facts, but they weren't therapeutic for their accuracy, were they?

With this person you might even want to keep them more in the loop than you normally might about "case conceptualization" and things of this nature, but not because she needs as many facts as possible about her life and psychological development; rather, because she needs someone to be absolutely straight with her. That is, she needs someone to *show her their mind* ever so freely, including their ideas about her, because what she *really needs* from another person is frankness, truth, and non-patronizing respect. Yet, these things cannot be delivered in words, or else we could just say to her, "I respect you in a non-patronizing way." This isn't how it works. It can only be shown. We need to have a handle on what to show, and when. To do it right, we somehow have to *contact* what people are, what they have been, and what they might be. And of crucial importance, it cannot be *mere facts* about someone's history (in this case, a very disturbed and controlling parent) that guides us. If we are responding to people in the right way, we are responding to something in real-time, something in the room that seeps into our consciousness to be acted upon (much more on that later).

A Call to Reject The World of Constructs

Once we see that there is no clear link between holding facts in our minds and fostering new thought, feeling, or behavior in another, we must wonder, however threatening, why we aim to teach people things? This is such a jarring proposition that many readers will refuse to take it seriously. But, please, let it jar you. Why are we always trying to transfer our expertise, our knowledge, and our information? Why do we associate the accumulation of empirical knowledge—and protocols *about* experience—with the improvement of experience? And why do we use artifacts of the construct world (e.g., treatment workbooks) to guide our interactions with people, when we have access to their real experience from the moment they sit down? There is an exceedingly strong argument that our intractable reverence for "knowing" grows from a dearth of humility and an arrogance of mind—and in part, it does. However, the better explanation has to do with fear. In our field, we have wished all of our knowledge, facts, and information out of their rightful place in the construct world and into the world of being—where they don't belong. We have done so because it is much easier on us.

The safety of preordained protocols is found in their distancing effect. In using them, the mind of the practitioner is, in effect, dissociated from *that which is* in the here-and-now. The alternative is making actual contact with the experience of the other, but doing so is fraught, dirty, and difficult. It also strips us of the professional garb we have come dressed in, and in an instant, *makes us human*—good!

It makes therapy a real relationship—good! It makes us real people, which is what *other* real people need—good! Despite whatever discomfort this can bring, it also happens to be necessary in helping people. To see facts as having primary, obvious, and undoubtable import in a therapeutic encounter, a meeting of two subjectivities, is the percept of constricted and fearful vision. Therapy as a fact-applying mission is a much easier and neater pursuit than entering the potential chaos and horror of all that is *this-ness* for the other; it's also far less useful.

To link simple cognitive learning with changes in behavior, improvements in well-being, and increased internal peace is profound misunderstanding. Facts might be true, but the truth of them yields them exactly no power to effect change in human beings. This is an inconvenient fact, and for the fact-obsessed, one that will not likely land. Psychotherapy is a pursuit to know people rightly, not to apply the facts that make us right.

Notes

1 Conscientiousness makes good clinicians, but sometimes those moved primarily by duty limit themselves in delving deeper into the patient's psyche. Being too responsible can inhibit openness to the other.
2 However, before reflexively agreeing that these concepts are meaningfully different (or meaningful at all), we'd do well to spend some time in the philosophical rabbit hole that, assuming we are thinking clearly, such terribly odd-sounding phrases evokes.

8

THE EXPERIENTIAL BASIS FOR RIGHT KNOWING

Love, Loss, and Loathing

This chapter will address the unknown: all that exists in the ocean of experience, which does not make its way into a particular person's experiential current, all the subjectivity that is out there to be had that does not make its way into one's subjective life. As laid out previously, what can and cannot be "be-d" in the domain of experience determines what can and cannot be known in the domain of cognition; thus, the unknown is something more than just "information about the world that we have yet to acquire." The deepest, most eternal meaning of the unknown is *all we cannot be that we really are*. Recall Harry. He cannot *be deserving*. He *knows* that "being deserving" is a state of being that exists but knowing so in his mind has never been the problem. He's always been able to know it; he's just never been able to be it. The all-important clinical question, then, which we will explore in this chapter is, "what is this *can't* about? *Why* can't he be it? Why is it *really* that people *can't* be what they *can't* be? What is the obstruction? What limits our personal "being repertoires?"

Being Repertoires

Consider a man whose capacity for aggression stops at thinking an unkind thought, and whose mind works a bit slowly. He might never *be funny* on his feet in the way a standup comic can be. And right out of the gate, we might grant that this limitation is somewhat determined (or at least informed) by biology. Nonetheless, we can never know the *true range* of his being repertoire until he devotes energy to expanding it. Sure, he (and much of his family) might lack the appropriate temperament and processing speed for witty humor (biological factors), but there might be equally obstructive, non-biological factors in the way— namely, the investments he has made in who he is,[1] which are not made from the

DOI: 10.4324/9781003305286-12

stuff of biological material, or from observable stuff at all. What if important relationships have moved this person, as a means of sparing love itself, to be accommodating, agreeable, and socially muted? This might put joking around out of reach so-to-speak, since it requires a kind of assertive energy, and can even bring with it interpersonal friction.

Were this the case, the obstruction to embodying funniness would not be a mere matter of his biological capacity, as subjectivity would have been cut with an injunctive. There would be a *prohibition* against funniness, *in being.* Yet he would not necessarily experience the force of prohibition: he wouldn't necessarily feel that funniness *shouldn't* be. He would only necessarily feel that it isn't: that it isn't part of his being. He might be aware, cognitively, that he has a hard time with humor, but he cannot be "aware" of the intrinsic processes that have limited his repertoire, since the investing process is not of mind; nor can he be aware of what being funny *is like*, even if he can conceptualize funniness. From within any given experiential current, this is the meaning of the rest of the ocean. It's unknown precisely because, in effect, it isn't there. Even if, cognitively, it can be characterized as "lacking," as *unelaborated being* goes, it is nothing of the sort. In being, it isn't missing; it just isn't.

When considered as an empirical variable, this outcome, "the absence of humor," might be a product of several predictor variables, both biological and environmental. However, from within the realm of conscious experience, these abstractions mean little. There, it *just simply is*: in his given, subjective experience, being humorless is true in a way that is *non-derivative*. This is essential to understand. The experience of humorlessness is not constructed from anything because it is not constructed at all. It is part and parcel of being itself. For him, it simply doesn't exist as part of self, where self is defined by those qualities of experience that fall within the bounds of normative consciousness; just as "I am from Savannah, GA" would not exist as part of self, were he from Dublin, where self is defined by one's propositionally derived self-concept.

In fact, funniness might be even more excluded from his *being* than Savannah from his *self-concept*. This is because conjuring to mind *the fact* of one's hometown requires additional steps that the *experience* of humorlessness doesn't. The latter isn't a fact; it's something that is altogether known in the absence of cognitive elaboration, or perhaps prior to it. As it exists in *this-ness*, not the cognitive elaboration thereof, the man is contacting it all the time; he *is it*—being it, living it, all the time. Whereas knowing of his hometown requires at least some cognition, if only the automaticity of declarative memory, knowing of his lack of humor does not. His lack of humor is not conceptual. It is only made conceptual through characterizing it, which means, as odd as it sounds, it is even *more real* than the fact that he is "from Ireland" because it is somehow more given. Stranger still, even if he is aware of his humorlessness, in its propositional form (i.e., "I'm not funny"), its truth is somehow diluted. As he "knows" it free of cognition, couching it in cognition adulterates its true essence, which is in being "be-d"—rather than being thought.

Maybe this man's non-funniness cannot be changed. After all, surely there are immutable aspects of being, given to us by non-negotiable factors like genes. But here is the question I want to pose: how would we distinguish between the human outcomes that are truly fixed by biology and those that only seem so? Could some of our apparently unalterable traits be attributable to the ineffable process by which people make investments in their own being? But this raises another problem. If there is such a process as, mustn't *it* be governed by biology? For that matter, mustn't biology rest at the bottom of every human outcome? Yes, if you ask modern man, but he is often too sure of himself—and his certitude ought to compromise his credibility.

What is Body and Mind?

In 2022 we aren't sure what we mean by body and mind. We do know that distinct thoughts, feelings, and behaviors maintain distinct biological correlates. For example, anger looks like a different thing, physiologically speaking, than sadness; that is, it registers differently in terms of fMRI activity and blood pressure. However, the fact that thought, feeling, and behavior is amenable to biological description need not mean that biology represents the bottom most layer and ultimate driver of each; nor does it mean that physiology is the criterion for what is "really going on" with someone. Yet, from our model of the world, we wonder why someone is confused and paranoid, only until we learn that their "dopamine production is out of control." Then we think, satisfied, "oh, they have schizophrenia."

At the same time, however, we seem also to be overcoming our "physiology first" ethos. In claiming a mind-body connection, we seem to be endorsing the idea that biological factors are not so fixed as to determine human life and are perhaps even influenced by factors less physical in nature. We have found, for example, that what we call, *being angry*, seems a contributor to heart disease; and that what we call, *being negativistic*, seems a contributor to the development of cancer. These paths to disease are quite different than eating too much steak or smoking too many Marlboros in that they include "mind processes." In light of such findings, we proclaim that the body is impacted by the mind, and that no human outcome is the simple product of observable cellular activity; to the contrary, the mind—whatever that means—has its own effect on cellular phenomena, so we claim. And this seems to be true. What we call "body" and what we call "mind" certainly seem to impact each other.

What goes unnoticed, however, is that we are saying contradictory things. First, we say there are two systems (i.e., mind and body), which chronically overlap, influence each other, and work in tandem; soon thereafter, however, we claim that these two systems are really *only one system* (i.e., "mind-body"). So, what do we really think? In contemporary research, where mind and body must be made separate categories in order to be examined, dualistic models are prevalent, even if only implicitly, despite that we claim them to be increasingly out of fashion. Whatever we claim, we operate as if the brain accounts for mostly everything. This is readily seen in a common confusion that brain processes *cause* all other phenomena (e.g., emotional and behavioral), even those with which they could only possibly be correlated (not to mention in the view that the brain *causes* consciousness itself, despite that no observable bridge connects the two). The brain, while a very important organ to understand, is an organ, nonetheless. It is body, nonetheless.

Consider the finding that "gratitude," as assessed, defined, and measured by way of its biological correlates, tends to reduce "distress" as assessed, defined, and measured by way of its biological correlates. This finding could be pointed to as evidence that body phenomena (i.e., physiological markers of distress) are impacted by mind phenomena (i.e., the cognitive and emotional state of gratitude). Studies like these show that one thing impacts the other and seem to reveal a mind-body relationship—and in some sense, they do. But let's look closer at this variable, gratitude. It seems that its existence is owed precisely to its manifestations in the physical body as well as its amenability to physiological description. That is, despite sounding like a state of mind, this hypothetical study makes gratitude, functionally speaking, into a biological algorithm—one that might be associated with certain behavior from oxytocin and other hormones, and other very specific brain activity.

Psychological variables defined by biological activity cast doubt on our commitment to mind and body. When the "mind-stuff" that we so fervently claim impacts "body-stuff" is couched, confirmed, and tracked biologically, what could we possibly mean when we say it's mind stuff? It seems that we mean it is less visible (e.g., a cardiac patient's "over-controlled anger" is a murkier variable and harder to see than any of the chemicals contained in his cigarettes, making it, in our paradigm, a mind-related precursor to heart problems). Yet, as empirical inquiry goes, we tend to know both of them by way of—that is, we tend to use as their validity criterion—bodily processes. This is not to say that all studies put psychic factors in terms of body, but all studies that do so seem to have the most clout (and perhaps receive the most funding) because our "truth serum view" (i.e., our *actual* view) is that mind processes *most exist* (i.e., are most validated) when they reliably co-occur with body processes. For example, anger is *really* anger when it is correlated with rising blood pressure; and schizophrenia is *really* schizophrenia when it is associated with excess dopamine. This practice certainly doesn't obstruct us from evermore facts; it only betrays that our loyalties lie with the body, no matter what kind of lip service we pay to mind.

From this perspective, our empirically derived relationships between mind and body (e.g., between *anger* and *cardiac problems*) are better cast as relationships between brain and body (e.g., between *anger defined by its associated brain phenomena* and *cardiac problems*), which means our mind-body claims disappear into body-body claims. It appears we have found innumerable body-body connections, only to have mischaracterized them. Outside of the language we use to differentiate things we can see with our eyes from things we cannot, the notion of "mind versus body," as we currently construe it, references a distinction with no difference. There is only body.

Where is our Mind?

This is the fate of every "mind variable" whose biological correlates are sought, since finding them quietly transforms it into the stuff of body. What's more, conceiving of every human phenomenon as its brain-situated corollary is a trend that results in the exile of all that is unverifiable with brain. This is a problem, though, because as a means of representing actual human experience, the brain is a blunt tool. For example, feelings of contentment and fear can be distinguished on fMRIs, but would such a machine register differently the satisfaction brought about by your favorite food versus an impending vacation versus an achievement at work? Maybe eventually our machines will pay attention to every qualitative nuance contained in human experience, but as for now, they cannot even be seen (certainly not all of them). But the utility of our machines is less a problem than our reverence for them. We are overjoyed with technology that presses real human experience into a caricature of itself in the form of neural activity. This speaks to our loss of humanity, discussed in the Introduction of this book. My point is not that brain research is unhelpful (in certain ways, it definitely is). My point is to show what modern people, including many in mental health, really think of humanity.

At present, we are aiming to understand life from the inside of a closed circuit, and we seem not to know it. When all our knowledge about mind and body (e.g., gratitude reduces distress; anger worsens hearts) is finally describable in biological terms, we will have lost our way. We will then be committed to circularity, since the whole of scientific discourse about mind and body will take place vis-à-vis the body. We are headed in this direction now, and we will only gain speed as we knight the brain, an organ, as the arbiter of what's *really* going on. Our discussion of people, at every point, will be contained within and attached to the body. Consider that someone, in 2022, could explain their affinity for charity in the following way:

> "When exposed to the right stimulus, my brain undergoes chemical changes that result in associated states of positive emotion, especially thankfulness, which has clear neurological correlates and results in my behavioral activation system being induced, chemically speaking, into prosocial behavior, which also maintains correlating brain activity."

While this statement might be technically true, there is no mind in sight, or at least there need not be. The entirety of the process, from start to finish, can be explained in terms of the body—it is a biological sequence. Sure, some of our words sound like mind words, but all of them are situated, by one process or another, in the body. This statement is thus not one as to *how the mind impacts the body*; rather, it is a statement *that the body impacts the body*. It is a description of how the body works, albeit a very intricate one. If there was even one step in the course of a given "mind-body" mechanism to which the body were not attached—i.e., one phenomenon that was not situated in or validated by the body—things would be different. Then, mind itself would be involved as an independent thing. And in turn, body processes could be in fact attributed to something other than themselves. Currently, body processes cannot be attributed to anything other than themselves because mind processes, which are the only real candidates, at bottom, are nothing but other body processes.

"How do the mind and body work together," we ask, to which we reply, "the body works *so complexly*." We can't get out of the body circuit, and thereby make our explanations *actual explanation* for how mind impacts body, without referring to something non-body. Imagine a student asks a teacher, "How does the mind work as a contributor to Bodily Process A," to which the teacher replies, "by way of bodily Processes B, C, and D." In effect, the teacher would be saying, "the body *also* works in these ways." This is no explanation of how something *other than body* influences Bodily Process A. It cannot be since every construct, process, and variable *involved in explaining* exists as a function of the body circuit, whether they are contained within the body (i.e., pure body variables) or attached to the body (body variables we call mind variables but prefer to validate via the brain, like gratitude). And so, the explanation depends fully on the body.

Where We're Headed: Human Being as Human Brain

Down the road, when all variables, psychic or otherwise, have brain-based algorithms and analogues, we will know much less than we will be convinced we do. We will say we have a mind-body paradigm, about which we know a lot, but in explaining what causes it to work in the way it does, we will be fated to invoke *only body*. This will have to be the case if all our variables maintain body coefficients, if each of them is a mere consequence—a mere appendage—of observable neurological processes. What we end up with in that situation is "human being as human brain."

Such a situation would be helped by humility. We simply might not yet understand what consciousness is, what it contains, and how it brings into observability and knowability that which it does. This is not our working assumption at present. We believe that *"everything that is"* can be brought into description with the right tools. But we might be wrong. This does not mean that consciousness houses strange forces of which we cannot know anything and which maintain control over all aspects of human life. It only means that an honest observer could conclude that popular attributions of body processes to mind processes are in fact attributions of body processes to other kinds of body processes; and, thus, while our instinct to connect the body with something less physical than itself is perfectly natural, right, and a true read of human consciousness, we might also be wholly unprepared—and much too pleased with our powers of observation—to grip what this might actually mean.

There might be plenty of human processes that contribute to the way our bodies and brains work, which exist beyond observation, thereby ruling themselves out, at least at present, as conceptualizable, mechanizable, or even *knowable*. Simply, aspects of ourselves that we cannot observe nor formulate might impact those aspects of ourselves that we can. Thus, it could be that physical processes are impacted by something less physical than them; but it might also be that our working conceptualization of what "non-physical" means, no matter how developed we take it to be, is a misunderstanding (or an early understanding, more sympathetically). And when understanding is in its infancy, it's wiser to leave possibilities open, rather than shut them: we human beings might well be more than the components of ourselves that we can observe and situate in language. In short, we human beings might be the mysteries we seem to be.

Back to Being

Now, why does all of this matter to the question posed above: "what prevents people from *being new things*?" It matters because it might mean that the *experiences of self in which people invest,* which are not the stuff of the physical world and which refuse observation and conceptualization as we know them (regardless of my naming them in this book[2]), could contribute to many more human processes than we think. They could even contribute to the way one's physiology works.

If this were the case, our being repertoires (e.g., relative humor–humorlessness), which are thought to be constrained by biology, might be somewhat less constrained than we generally think. Am I claiming that by revising the experiences of self in which one is invested could cause them grow three inches taller at age 40? Hardly—I am proposing that while our being repertoires are obviously set by biology to some extent, we do not really know how set they are because we do not fully know how *our investments in particular experiences of self* influence the physical (physiological) world. And technically speaking, this is not something we can know. Any research paradigm that operationalizes "experiences of self" is claiming to have observed and conceptualized that of which cognition knowns nothing. No representation *is* one's real experience of self; all are knockoffs.

All of this means that biology might not be the deepest *can't* with respect to why people *can't* be new things. Something more essential might be informing biology, something we will never find in our elaborate systems. There might be a deeper-seated, more precious *can't*, which has to do with the investing process by which certain qualities of consciousness become us. To freely and openly wonder why people can't be what they can't be, I think we have to grant our love-sparing investments—those that have created the experience of self that grips us—exponentially more due than our intellects are generally prepared to. I think we have to uncorrupt ourselves.

Right, Wrong, and Love: Morality Striving in A Different Key

Recall from Chapter 6 that people invest in the experience of self they do precisely because it spares love. Being one thing and not another (or some things and not others) safeguards love as a potential in the world. For Harry, the experience of "underserving-ness" was a better route than that of "deserving-ness" insofar as the former prevented his situation from registering as completely loveless. As he came to experience himself as undeserving, failing to receive love became reasonable, which made his situation unremarkable; in turn, love had not done him wrong and therefore warranted no criticism, rage, nor renunciation. This is why the experience of self in which he invested could be said to have saved love: it caused love to go unscathed. From this angle, no matter how distorted it might be, all the mental activity that both *grows from* and is meant to *engender* this same experience of himself could be thought of as his attempt to keep love in the world: it induces the experience of self that makes love—and the prospect that he might still receive it—possible. However paradoxical, Harry's entire pursuit to experience himself as undeserving is the pursuit of love. But it's also more than that.

Remembering from Chapter 6 that being loved *means* one's morality, all the perceptual, cognitive, and behavioral processes aimed at engendering the *experience of self* that ensures one might still be loved, represent *more than just* attempts to spare love; to the extent that one's suitability for love *means* one's morality, all of these processes, as they are meant to occasion love, are quietly meant to *make one good*. All of these processes, which together constitute people themselves, must also represent *morality striving*. Applying this formula to certain cases can seem bizarre (and even offensive), so let's start with an uncontroversial application.

Imagine a young girl raised with disinterested caregivers, dismissive peers, aloof teachers, but endowed with a good dose of natural competency. In words, her intrinsic investments might yield an experience of herself as "wholly self-sufficient" (an investment that spares love via negating all the harm of neglect). From that starting point, her life would come to have all the trappings of conventional decency. She would work to no end, become very educated, save money, and value personal responsibility highly, at times frighteningly so. She would always appear to be "doing right." To anyone paying attention, her entire life would read like something straight from the "traditional morality playbook." Her "experience of self" and every perceptual, cognitive, and behavioral process *meant to induce it* (her way of seeing, thinking, and behaving) appears to any half-reasonable, culturally embedded observer, as bona-fide morality-striving.

Now for a harder case. Consider a man who grew up in a situation that caused an investment in "self as hostile." Maybe this came about as his loved ones ridiculed his inability to stand up for himself, or because his rough neighborhood allowed for affiliation only through aggression and cruelty. Whatever the circumstances, the part of him tracking the relative presence of love noted that love is simply more available when people are tough, strong, mean. If at 17, he beats someone half-to-death in a bar for spilling his drink, engages in orchestrated crime throughout his 30s, and settles down at 45, only to treat his own family terribly, we would not reflexively characterize his life as an attempt to be *good*. In fact, regarding his manifest behavior in the world, we might see *none of it* as morality striving.

However, is there a way that his behavior could be interpreted as an attempt to be good? This is a terrible question for the position in which it puts the answerer. To say "yes" seems to endorse an upside-down ethical system. Yet, saying "no" is not only mistaken; it is to render oneself completely useless if tasked with helping him. However difficult or destructive, his preferred experience of self, from which his mental activity and behavior grow, is the product of a quiet, unwitting love calculus. Strange as it sounds, how one is in the world is inherently morality-seeking, where one's own morality—one's own goodness—is attained through achieving the experience of self that has become silently associated with love. Note that this formula places no constraints on what that "experience of self" might be.

The investments people make in themselves as a means of saving love need not translate into thought, feeling, or behavior that is manifestly good, proper, or right (this is not to say these concepts mean nothing—they most certainly do). It need only translate into thought, feeling, and behavior that *feels right*. And what does it mean for certain thought, feeling, and behavior to feel right? It means only that it puts one in contact with a familiar experience of self, one meant to keep love—*and thereby one's own goodness*—within reach.

For the woman above, her preferred experience of self (i.e., self as self-sufficient) happens to align perfectly with the values that surround her. Assuming she lives in the West, being self-sufficient *is* being good, at least arguably (for better or worse). This is why, with no problem, we see her way of being as morality striving. But if we looked harder, we could see this very thing in everyone's way of being. She, nor the violent man above, are out to satisfy any ethical system external to them (and even if they are, there is another "system" equally or more important to them). Both are out to satisfy the experience of self that means their own goodness, by meaning that love might exist for them.

If you were trapped in a burning building, it would feel right to move toward more oxygenated rooms because you know, innately, that without oxygen, life cannot be lived. We don't go around talking about it in this way because we are sophisticated and cell-based in our explanations of people, but watch closely. Inevitably, the trajectory on which you find someone, in some way or another, means to them, breathable air. For some, total interpersonal withdrawal is oxygen, for others altruism is, and for still others, total hostility is. Any thought, feeling, or action can feel right, so long as it engenders the experience of self one is invested in being. This is the case regardless of the relative rightness-wrongness we might assign to any thought, feeling, or action from within any one of our cognitively elaborated (and very real) ethical systems. This in no way means our tough guy from above, for example, isn't responsible for all of his behavior. To the most exceptional contrary, he is unambiguously responsible for every drop of it—and good therapy will place this burden lovingly but squarely on his shoulders. His problem, however, is not fundamentally about conduct; it is fundamentally about love, as all human problems are.

A Humane View of Psychopathology: Old Waters, New Waters, and Symptoms

When people find themselves at the outermost boundary of their experiential currents, uncomfortable with nearby and unknown waters, their sense of their own goodness is under assault. In turn, perceptual, cognitive, and behavioral processes unfold that ensure experience remains what experience has always been, that *they* remain what they have always been—thereby providing stabilization. These processes can often yield what looks like simple misperception from the outside, and maybe it is misperception, but for the (mis)perceiver, the benefit is worth the cost.

Imagine someone who becomes paranoid about her boss' intentions in the very same moment she is offered a life-changing promotion. To her coworkers, this might seem odd. They might think that her mind is not working properly, that she must be "misconstruing reality" to become agitated and fearful over such an "objectively good thing." But what if we knew that experiencing herself as valuable and successful ran counter to that which she is most invested in being; that, for her, part of being moral—part of *being good enough for love*—involves *being inferior*. Then, we could understand why she construes a well-deserved promotion from a competent boss who is happy about her work as an "undeserved promotion from a know-nothing boss who is promoting her for some unknown reason, obviously unrelated to merit."

Her striving mind, entirely "in the tank" for her needed experience of self, delivers her to a paranoid perspective, but it also spares her an experiential encounter with the waters beyond her current. By way of paranoia, her mind fights off a new and emerging experience of herself (i.e., self as valuable); in turn, she is able to remain in her much-needed experiential current (i.e., self as inferior). The paranoia, though terrible, is less terrible than adopting a new kind of self, one that threatens love, and thereby her own goodness.

Next, imagine a man whose mind strives toward construing the world in a way that generates within him an experience of specialness (he is intrinsically invested in "self as special"); now imagine that he is fired on Friday, broken up with on Saturday, only to find himself on a train headed to the unemployment office on

Monday morning. His fellow passengers are reading their emails, worrying about their families, and generally focusing on themselves, as people on trains do. When it becomes evident to him that nobody is paying him much attention, a stark feeling of "normalcy" begins to set in. There he is, approaching the perimeter of his current, not yet in unknown waters, when he becomes abruptly hostile toward everyone on the train. He suddenly finds them to be staring at him incessantly; they even seem overly curious about what he is thinking. This "brief psychotic episode" (in DSM lingo) seems to have materialized out of the clear blue sky. But maybe it didn't. Maybe in the underlying, intrinsic world, he was approaching a threatening experience of self (in words, "self as normal"), when his cognition suddenly created a scene in which he was, once again, at the center of it all. Was it uncomfortable? Yes, delusions of persecution and intrusion are painful experiences. Did it spare him? Yes, it allowed him to retain the experience of self that is most familiar and most stabilizing.

Because our taken for granted experiential currents have been constructed as a means of maintaining contact with love, the waters beyond them (i.e., new experiences of self) mean psychic havoc. They first mean loss. Should we wade into new waters, the experience of self we most associate with love is no more. In addition to loss, new, unknown waters also mean antipathy. When our current modes of being are meant to retain love, and our attempts to remain situated in them therefore mean morality-striving, however ill-conceived our current modes of being seem from the outside, alternative ones, *to us*, are more than just different. They are worse, even morally deficient. This is true, regardless of their ingredients. Whether someone is struggling with emergent experiences of tranquility or hostility, success or failure, vibrancy or lethargy, that which one is *reluctant to be* threatens a silent, unconceptualizable value system: one made not of reason, deliberative contemplation, or concepts but of the experiences of self that mean love, and thereby one's own goodness.

From this view, the barrier to new ways of being is quite simple, and its simplicity is trumped only by its power. The waters surrounding each of our currents, though they hold the promise of new ways of being, also promise trouble. First, they ensure the *fear, grief, and loss* associated with moving away, psychically speaking, from love; and second, they ensure *self-directed hate*, the kind we reserve for people too contemptible for love, which is exactly who we would be, should we violate our love ensuring—and thereby goodness ensuring—experiences of self. Thus, the waters just beyond the perimeter of our experiential currents, in every direction, are infested with loss and loathing.

Beyond Circumstance: A Foundational Human Problem

Because being differently, even in the most useful and mature ways, jeopardizes love, it also destabilizes people. From the viewpoint I am offering, psychological symptoms are still real, valid, and correlated with observable processes in brain and body; however, at a deeper level, they are the consequence of a person contending with something in the intrinsic world—in particular, newly emerging "experiences of self," which people will be called on to embody just by virtue of being alive.

From this lens, the foundational problem, the one we all share, is not psychiatric but human. That which we are invested in being (e.g., powerful) will inevitably clash with that which really and truly materializes in being (e.g., weak). Psychological development, then, is the coming to terms with one's own humanity, certain components of which are more or less difficult, depending on one's investments. If any one of us is to live peacefully, we are required to give up our preferred modes of being for being itself, for the ocean itself, which does not kowtow to the investments we have made in what being ought to be and is instead ruled by what being actually *is*. And what is being? What is every human being, all the time? We are every possible experience of self—nothing less. Our currents, whatever they look like, are for the birds. We, you and I, are the ocean.

For all of the truly unavoidable pain that human life holds for us, at the bottom of all suffering is something inconceivably simple: oneself as one is. The self we prefer, cherish, and cling to will disappear and be replaced by something that frightens and offends us. The universal obstruction to the adoption of new experiences of self is the loss and offense caused by that which we might otherwise be, which is only another way of saying, that which we *really are*. We all must grow our capacity and willingness to welcome everything we already are, always have been, and always will be.

The purpose of therapy, then, is to enact a method of knowing people that helps them to be all they might be, good and bad. It is a method of helping people to move toward the truths of experience; first, the truths of theirs, but then, the truths of experience at large—all of it—with less heartache and hate, with less suffering. Ultimately, good therapy targets the dilemma at the core of all other dilemmas, which is simple and goes like this: while there is certainly a brand of human suffering that comes about because of our inability to *bear the world* wherein we find ourselves, the worst kind of human suffering comes about because the world wherein we find ourselves is not one in which we can *bear ourselves*.

Knowing Someone Rightly: The Expansion of Being Repertoires

People often say they have sought therapy due to discomfort or distress. What they almost never say is that they feel far from love. But they do. New experiences of self threaten to eviscerate the potential for love as one knows it, via threatening the mode of being that makes one good enough to acquire it. What we know of anyone seeking therapy is that something intolerable in being, some this-ness (self as "X" or "Y"), has materialized or threatens to. Maybe a promotion has made them feel more competent than they *can be*, or maybe a thankless job has made them less unique than they *can be*. Underneath all identifiable "symptoms," there is a refused experience of self. Yet, whatever experience of oneself is being kept at bay, it is as much a part of human life as any other, regardless of the notion of self that occupies that person's cognitively constructed identity.

It is essential to note that we need not make conscious calculations about the meaning of this or that experience of self emerging or not emerging from within the intrinsic world. Rather, somewhere very deep, we know when consciousness is threatening to make itself over; we know when we are close to the edge of our current; and we respond, unknowingly, to prevent an encounter with a new experience of self (i.e., new qualities of consciousness). Symptoms, *which have never set in by conscious volition*, achieve this. No one has ever said to themselves: "I am not invested in experiencing myself as lonely; therefore, I will keep my emerging, genuine, and natural experience of loneliness (a new experience of self) at bay, by instead experiencing a numb depression for 18 months."

This is why symptoms arise in such a way that can often seem to make little sense, at least when run through our cognitive apparatuses, and why we can't always find their "antecedents." The experiences of ourselves we reject for their promise to induce loss and loathing exist only in the world of being. We cannot conceive of them, not fully. Some part of us simply knows that we will soon bump into something unpleasant or that we already have; in turn, symptoms emerge. Although everyone has their recurrent brand of them, any symptoms can serve as a barricade to a new self—and all of them do. Symptoms materialize when a non-invested in (and non-preferred) experiences of self is on the horizon.

Knowing another in the right way is nothing like a protocol. It is an approach to being, one I will further describe down the road. What I want to say about it here is that it targets the most common but most profound human problem: it helps people bear all they might be. Ultimately, the best psychotherapies instill in people a sense that perhaps they could *be differently, be more*—and *still be*. When carried out in good faith, something amazing happens. Sometimes over time and sometimes so abruptly as to jar everyone watching, the parameters of a person's being repertoire simply expand. Returning to the beginning of the chapter, from growth in one's *experience of self*, which is not of a material nature, often come changes in processes that once seemed wholly governed by biological material. People who seemed temperamentally, slow, pessimistic, or even humorless can *just simply* change; they can *just simply* discover modes of experience once assumed to be obstructed by physiological factors.

When known in the right way, people's experience changes, eventually for the better; but first and more importantly, for the truer. Right knowing is right because it neutralizes the loss, loathing, and more, that comes with being new things—things we most certainly are. It permits the other to abandon the current in favor of the ocean, thereby granting themselves significantly more flexibility in being. This kind of freedom has many benefits, but the most important one—and there's no close second—is a newfound freedom to be ethical.

Notes

1 This phrase, "investments in who one is," is a reference to the investing process discussed in both the Introduction and Chapter 6. Automatically and unwittingly, we make investments in those "experiences of self" that some non-cognitively situated part of us has deemed will spare love (to be abbreviated as "the investing process").

2 Remember that one's "experience of self" defies conceptualization. Even calling "it" that doesn't capture but overshoots the mark.

9

A SHRINKING SELF IS A GROWING SELF

Because people enter it for so many different reasons, psychotherapy is a pursuit that could be said to have infinite tasks. Pragmatism thus must be part of the clinician's personality; if it isn't, the real-world problems patients most care about might never be solved. An unpredictable chunk of any given therapy session might therefore consist of a collaborative attempt to find solutions to any of life's many complications. However, while concrete problems will be addressed head-on in any worthwhile psychotherapy, the deepest goal of the therapeutic encounter is not the improvement of circumstances. In fact, a therapy process that has become one grand effort to rearrange the external world can begin to feel like a tired game of whack-a-mole, wherein one problem after another is "fixed" yet somehow nothing changes.

More than circumstance, the target of psychotherapy is simply subjectivity as one knows it (i.e., as one experiences it). Changes that happen here hold more power to cultivate a peaceful internal world than do any modifications to the conditions of the outer world. This chapter will not directly describe how psychotherapy can facilitate such improvements (as the following two chapters will). Rather, it will lay out what is arguably the most important consequence of internal change: becoming more ethical and more humane. Such a shift can take place within any one of us, thereby changing the external world as any of us knows it.

The Terms of Existence

To whatever extent human problems cannot be changed, any good therapist is some part philosophical quietist insofar as they help patients to see old problems as non-problems, thereby affording people more tranquility. Hiding in every

DOI: 10.4324/9781003305286-13

model of psychotherapy is a related assumption: distress and its solutions are as constituted in how one orients to life as they are in the events of life themselves. For example, therapy cannot erase a terrible memory of being abused or abusive, nor can it bring back to life the people most precious to us. Yet sitting in a room for one to two hours per week, talking, somehow reduces the intensity of the pain surrounding real historical events, despite lacking an ounce of potential to alter them.

As the harshness of existence will find everyone, it must be true that the manner in which we relate to its rather unforgiving parameters is our very first problem, a more important problem than the parameters themselves because the parameters *just are*. To be *truly* on the side of another person, we must view them as possessing the capacity to live well *despite*, to live well *with a lack*, and to live well *anyway*. Believing that living is something other than this might only mean that one has not yet lived long enough to know otherwise. And we should be kind to people like this, for our frustration with their naivete might only be envy on masquerade. Some part of everyone wishes to be so childlike.

What I am suggesting can be a hard pill for many in the modern world, perhaps especially therapists whose major identification is that of "scientist." All of our cleverness, all of our methods and tools and facts, have fooled many into the illusion that human problems exist precisely to be toppled, that our intellectual and moral prowess will continue to barrel toward every human problem at record speed, only to eventually eradicate every last one. This is precisely what we are saying when we say that certain variants of human suffering, all of which are as old as time even if they've not always had technical names (e.g., "recurrent, moderate depression"), can be "cleared up" in eight quick sessions. From this fantastical world view, human strife is a nuisance to be resolved, even done away with entirely. Lucky for us, some human trouble is fixable; but the kind with unreserved potential to destroy people isn't. This kind is exclusively endurable; harder still, if one wants a reasonably satisfying life, it must be endured. The closer we come to claiming that all human suffering can be targeted and removed in the same way a tumor might be, the more readily we betray our total naivete with respect to the complexities, sensitivities, and difficulties of being a person; worse still, the more readily we betray our disrespect for what it means to be a struggling person, which, in no uncertain terms, is precisely what it means to be a person, *period*. To entertain the idea that all psychic struggle is subject to cure with just the right set of therapeutic techniques is not simple academic ambition; it is a failure of empathy so astoundingly profound as to teeter on the verge of psychopathic cruelty.

Each of us must contend with losing every single thing we have ever cared about; each of us will confront our own death and the death of those we would never choose to live without; each of us will confront our ever-growing physical and mental deterioration, and that of others, some of whom were represented as "invincible" in concepts, until our senses showed us otherwise; and each of us will hear, to varying degrees of chronicity, the low hum of doubt, loneliness, and sadness. What's more, as we take action in our lives, aiming for one thing or another, we can't really know if it's "right"—not objectively so—but we must continue to do, nonetheless (Chapter 4). And as we continue to move forward, we need to construe every step as valuable, even if it proves not to be, lest we might just *stop doing* altogether, which is only appealing until one tries it. These are realities that will not be soothed by the behavioral technologies of clinical psychology, the material technologies of Silicon Valley, or the sociopolitical technologies of any governing class.

We can be sure, then, that any instinct to resolve the very conditions of our humanity, to the extent it is aimed outward, is an illusion. For the pain of being human, no medicine will be found in the external, the material, or the worldly; when we need soothing and look to such things, we will find temporary bursts of peace, but to the degree we mistake them for genuine cure, we have only mis-judged the shape of the material world. In time it will again show itself as a circle, and the position we have deemed special or ultimate will show itself as just another point along its circumference. Our notable contentment will surely fade because the world to which we are magnetized for answers—the one around us—contains none that can last. The one within us, however, was made to yield the most important kind of contentment—*contentment, despite*. Alternative, exter-nally derived kinds of contentment are fantasies; anyone pretending they aren't, whether a technologist or psychologist, is doing a disservice to the people for whom they are pretending. Psychotherapists, especially, must be as *real* as they are *optimistic*. Nothing but equal proportions will do.

The Problem with Problem-Solving the World

I once listened to a clinician describe her frustration with feeling unable to help her patient. She was seeing a woman who, weeks before, lost her husband in a terrorist attack. This therapist was in the market for "better interventions," and hoping that her fellow clinicians would be selling some. She seemed to believe, somewhere deep down, that with the right "protocol" or "intervention," she might help to evaporate a kind of agony by which any person could easily be ruined. The chasm between she and her patient was so large that the dynamic would have been better billed as a pay-per-view boxing match, rather than a collaborative therapy session:

> "In one corner, a numb and grieving mother, now face-to-face with all of the bona-fide meaninglessness, misery, and torment that human existence can viciously rain down on a person; and in the other corner, a devout empiricist and clinician, armed to the teeth with the latest acronym for reducing 'grief behaviors' in twelve short sessions!"

The situation that had befallen her patient was one over which she, nor anyone, had any control. Recognizing it as such would have been an internal intervention on the part of the clinician; it would have helped her to see that she had run up against the limits of psychiatry, psychology, and institutions altogether. This was not a job for a protocol but for a person, and probably one who doesn't take darkness as a problem but as a feature of human experience. In situations where there is no light, the best thing to do, it seems to me, is to sit there with people—and be kind. When there's nothing that can be done, that's the only thing that can be done. I should say that despite my outrage—it should be called that because that's what it was—I also felt a lot of sympathy for this clinician (albeit, only after the meeting). Someone seemed to have convinced her that psychology's methods work on tormenting despair in the way that Tylenol works on headaches. I think she found herself in a moment of desperation as she was coming to realize that her patient's pain was beyond her influence.

This story is only one consequence of our field's shared and delusional self-conception as "the problem solvers of human misery." Thankfully, while none of us can be magical enough to remove all the problems from someone's life, all of us can be moral enough to be with them amid any one of them, which is very often the best thing to do despite the field's rabid impulse to "fix." Needless to say, this grieving mother wasn't there to be fixed, given that she wasn't broken; in that situation, there is no healthier response than being inconsolably distraught. The key is to see that she was not there to have her suffering removed, nor to be made brighter. She was there because she needed someone to sit beside her—in the darkness.

Let's further consider the merits of "problem solving." Imagine a patient arrives at an intake session and attributes her depressed mood and suicidal thinking to the fact that she was not admitted to any of the colleges to which she applied. As so-called problem solvers, we would simply survey the external world, find the obstruction to her internal peace, and move it aside. Maybe there was a problem in the quality of her college applications, or her interview skills, or her test-taking abilities—just like that, we have treatment goals.

But what if we run into another kind of problem? What if she was declined entry to college because she simply wasn't smart enough? The modern world finds hypotheses like this offensive due purely to arrogance and fear. The world used to be modest and brave enough to admit that each of us is limited in our own special ways and, unfortunately, none of us can do all we wish (this is why it was Derek Jeter, not me, playing shortstop all those years for the Yankees).

In the case of this patient, what if her grades and test scores are indicative of someone who is very unlikely to succeed, educationally? To make it worse, what if she was so deeply invested in her cognitive capacity (i.e., her intellectual competency), that all attempts to dissuade her from school, by friends or family alike, induced a storm of animosity. Is there a practical problem to be "solved" here? Ultimately, yes: there are ways to live a satisfying existence that are not so cognitively demanding. However, by suggesting them to our patient and thereby exhibiting our complete commitment to "problem solving," we would so too reveal our complete disregard for her personhood, our complete callousness. If her dreams are truly not a viable possibility, the work of grieving, not problem solving, must begin. This is a cruel task that existence has laid in front of us, but it must be carried out anyway because the only alternative is self-deceit, which over time not only causes more pain; it promises, like nothing else, to slaughter one's capacity to be ethical.

Self-Deceit

Regarding this patient, it is easy to imagine the pain that would grow from relinquishing her preferred experience of herself (in language: self as cerebral). What's harder to see is the pain that would grow from holding onto it. To the extent that any of us refuses a new and unwanted experience of self, problems are likely to invade our lives. In her case, she might spend five years unsuccessfully applying to schools, and another five grieving the loss of not getting in, only to look up and feel she has missed out on other things that might have satisfied her. Through self-deceit, she would have deprived herself of the real and actual good that really and actually exists for her.

More importantly, though, such self-deceit will compromise her ability to treat others well. This is an ethical dilemma of the most massive proportions, and one that confronts every one of us in each passing moment if we possess the courage to see it. When one aims to retain old experiences of self that have passed (or are simply out of operation, currently), one is prone to resentment, bitterness, and envy, directed especially at those more fortunate or in less pain. From this position, the world can quickly become comprised of two groups: people who "get everything they want" and "me." The patient above might treat poorly anyone who suggests to her more realistic paths, no matter how good their intentions. She could mistake the genuine concern of others for malevolent disrespect. If her illusion was strong enough, she could lump together all such people as too immoral, stupid, or incompetent to see her ability.

Only one thing can ward off these kinds of outcomes—the development of the most genuine respect for life's most devastating and omnipresent feature: loss. We must learn to practice giving up everything because, one day, we will have to. Anything that *is*, could one moment from now, *cease to be*. This is most apparent in terms of that which is external to us. For example, we will have to give up our first mitt, our favorite neighborhoods, and the best of times; worst of all, we will have to give up people. These aspects of life, brutal as they are, are built right in. What I want to now discuss is a kind of loss much more subtle, which reads to me as the seed of all relational warfare: the loss of preferred experiences of self.

Immoral Behavior Requires Self-Deceit: Pam

Imagine a girl who grows up feeling completely taken with her father. Let's call her Pam. From the time she is young, she misses him the moment he leaves for work, and she awaits his return all day; she studies extra hard solely to receive his praise; and she respects him deeply because, by all reasonable standards, he is a good person. She works hard in life in order to earn his respect and praise and continues to do so even long after he has died. Her insatiable drive to be respected by authority, which began in love, also makes her a de facto loyalist. Anywhere she works, she puts the organization ahead of herself. Her soul is made for the approving gaze of higher-ups.

As a consequence of hard work and dutiful if childlike obedience, Pam, a lawyer, manages to secure a highly sought-after management position at her firm. This is just what she wants. As she works her way up the organizational ladder, she is fulfilling her more or less unconscious objective to experience herself as "pleasing to authority." She appreciates that her subordinates seem to respect her, but her sincerest concerns lie precisely with how authority sees her. Things are going well when something suddenly happens out of the clear blue sky, shaking her at her core.

With no warning and without consulting her, higher-ups within the law firm make a decision about her position. They hire a co-manager. Now, she must share her role, the one that gratified her so deeply, with someone the higher-ups just plopped down in front of her. This person, let's call her Kim, reports to work one Monday, assuming that she is expected to be there, that her co-manager will offer her collegiality, and that she will be presumed to have good intentions.

But Kim runs into Pam, for whom basic decency proves challenging. While Kim is a kind and competent person who has made no attempt to harm anyone, Pam is outrightly disdainful. To observers, it seems almost out of Pam's hands to treat Kim well. She is instinctually hostile, like a lizard. She is consistently rude and devaluing toward Kim, especially when Kim isn't around, and always angry about her presence when she is. I should note that this story was relayed to me by an old patient (who wasn't "Pam" or "Kim"). From my old patient's view, Pam could not speak Kim's name without spite. The word "Kim" was uttered with disgust, whether saying "Kim doesn't know anything about our computer system" (as if any new employee would), or "Thanks, Kim, for bringing five pizzas to our staff meeting." Pam's disdain and apparent hatred for Kim became so manifest that my patient (their coworker) began to assume the two had some kind of history. People, *bright* people, wondered, "was Kim the one who ran over and killed Pam's dog last year?"

Nobody could blame Pam for her negative emotion, as there is no doubt that the higher-ups behaved disrespectfully toward her. If they thought a co-manager was needed, they certainly should have let her know so before hiring one. Yet, this alone cannot account for Pam's brazen malice for Kim, who made not a single attempt to harm her. That is, one thing doesn't warrant the other.

Here, Pam is displaying the most common type of interpersonal immorality, the formula for which goes something like this: if your treatment of another human being is determined primarily by the extent to which that person bolsters the sense of self in which you are most invested, you are fated to be an ethical nightmare on two legs. Why does Kim's kindness, competency, and basic humanity fail to earn her any decency from Pam? Why is there so little good in Kim, as Pam sees it? These questions have a very simple answer: because Kim represents a challenge to the *experience of self in* which Pam is most invested. The intrinsic quality of consciousness for which she is always on the hunt is an experience of self as "pleasing to authority." In order to ward off an experience of herself she cannot bear (i.e., unpleasing to authority), she feels uncontrollable and immediate aversion for the person (who appears to be) obstructing her from the one she cannot do without (i.e., pleasing to authority).

Those prone to this "disappointment turned malice" formula are also susceptible to its flipside. Whoever manages to fortify Pam's preferred experience of self will earn instantaneous fondness. They will be seen as virtuous and good. Unfortunately, the extent to which people agree with us, flatter us, or admire us, has no necessary bearing on the quality of their ethical behavior or their character. Someone who forgets this (or doesn't buy into it at all) might find great overlap in the people they take to be "good and ethical" and the people who regularly compliment their new socks. Ask yourself if there is a thing in the world less humane than evaluating the quality of another person as a matter of their propensity to keep you in your own good graces. This practice strips other people of their personhood, humanity, and autonomy, and makes them into mere pawns for one's own self-regulation and personal comfort.

Goodness, whatever we mean by it, is determined by whether people *are good*, not by whether people, through reinforcing our most comfortable experiences of self, make us *feel good*. These things are conflated, however, in a range of ways, some less harmful than others. Most of us are susceptible to thinking especially well of a person after he or she complements some smart thing we said at a meeting, or after they flatter our fashion sense. After something like this happens, feeling warmly toward them is hardly an interpersonal high crime. But it doesn't make any sense to link it with something about their ethics, morals, or character. While complements and flattery do not (necessarily) rule out the complementor as being good and ethical, such gestures on their own say nothing about a person's relative goodness. Why? Because, again, feeling good about ourselves, being liked, or being thought of positively, cannot possibly be an indicator that the person making us feel this way *is good*.

The reader might be thinking, "sure, but I don't find people who flatter me to be good in any important, *ethical sense*; I just find them jovial and good-natured." This might be true of how most people operate most of the time; for example, no clear-minded parent would believe that because a given coworker once flattered their new haircut, he or she would be a good candidate to babysit their newborn. But when we are recognized for things more important to us, things that speak to our deeper sense of identity (as it is experienced, not thought), we can lose the ability to make this kind of distinction. When recognized for those ways of being that comport with one's intrinsic investments—the way in which one *needs to be*—the person doing the recognizing is often taken as innately good and ethical, nearly automatically.

As a quick sidebar, this is why psychopaths have so much success in the world. They are more than superficially charming; they see into what people most need to be, then capitalize. Yet there is a specific group of people wholly unsusceptible to psychopathic charm (and psychopaths can spot them): those who understand ethical behavior as something different than, *even orthogonal to*, that behavior which tickles them (i.e., inflates their needed experience of self). Those who cannot distinguish these things will assuredly be duped by the charming and orchestrating swindler, who aims always to provide a quick shot in the arm to the egos of those people he is swindling, people who, through needing such a shot so desperately, become easy prey. To those needy for self-inflation, social grease and charm is often mistaken for something of value. The true psychopath, knowing this perhaps before anything else, sniffs out this need and targets those imprisoned by it.

If Pam were our patient, she might convey to us her conflicted feelings toward "the administration," but the real trouble is not contained in the actual, real-world event—her demotion; it's not even contained in the deep feelings of having failed her father—which would be no picnic. Pam's realest trouble is the nature of being itself. As laid out previously, simply through existing, each of us makes investments in what consciousness will be. From a whole ocean of them, we invest in specific qualities of experience as a means of retaining love. Pam only feels comfort, only feels acceptable to herself, when she experiences herself as pleasing to authority. Her trouble, like all of ours, is that the external world makes no promises to indulge or even safeguard the investments we have made in that which we will be. It doesn't matter which qualities of consciousness have become self; to understand reality is to understand that by virtue of having them, they are under threat, since a *shifting experience of oneself* is the indicator of existence itself.

Thus, no matter how frightening or comforting, no matter how predictable or surprising, changing experiences of self, in the broadest, most cosmic terms, are *a non-event*. Alternatively, they could be thought of as *a never-ending, chronic, ubiquitous event*, in the same way that something like breathing is. Existence has guaranteed that our most precious investments, those we have made in who we will be (i.e., self as *this-ness*) will be rattled, jarred, demolished, simply by being alive. At the center of life is not this self and the subjective quality of *this-ness* that goes with it, but loss of this self and ever-impending *that-ness*.

The Highest Deceit: The Most Intractable Self

As I write this, there is a story in the news about celebrities who bribed college officials in order to have their children admitted to the country's best schools.

Though this behavior represents a clear violation of basic ethics, from the perspective I am offering, it isn't driven purely by malice. It's much sadder than that. When someone is brittle with respect to the experiences of self they can bear, they become engaged in a destructive little game that has one goal: ward off every intolerable experience of self. The so-called "Varsity Blues" scandal is best explained not by the parents' greed or celebrity or entitlement, even if all such factors are in play. At the *causal* bottom of one's willingness to violate other people is nothing unique to the rich and influential but, simply, one's relationship with oneself. In the case of these parents, this relationship is exactly what it looks like. They would rather *be criminals* than *be someone* whose progeny is not sufficiently charmed (or doesn't *seem so*).

To be sure, there are times when the self, experienced as noxious, is meant to be altered. As examples, when we are sick, we aim to make ourselves well; when we are anxious in a crowd, we flee for comfort; and when life is difficult, however we might, we try to change it. In itself, a desire to improve the state in which one finds themselves cannot be thought of as immoral. What makes immorality is a person's willingness to alter a given experience of the self *at any cost*. If we were *willing to do anything* to become well, to leave the crowd, or to have a better life, immorality would be only a few strides away—wouldn't it?

Those who find that they would do anything to achieve a very specific experience of themselves (e.g., celebrities who can *only be special*; characters like Pam who *can only be respected*) have become unable to bear the huge majority of that which they are. In the worst cases, there is only one experience of themselves they can tolerate, which is to say, there is one self and one self only; and, damningly, it must be upheld at any cost. One's frequency of experiential discomfort is a direct consequence of the force with which one has intrinsically invested in *who they are*. When that which one *needs to be* is increasingly specific, normal life, which requires flexibility, will hold special power to destroy them; in turn, they will destroy others. This is the case for both Pam and the criminal parents mentioned above. Pam doesn't merely *prefer* to be respected; *being respected* is all she can be. The criminal parents don't merely *prefer* to be special people with special progeny; they can *only be special people with special offspring*.

Poor Conduct in a Different Light

The most superficial goal of poor conduct is to change the terms of the external world (e.g., to get one's daughter admitted to Yale through bribery). But in the final analysis, whether known to the perpetrator or not, all their poor conduct has a deeper aim: to right the terms of their internal world. From this lens, unethical behavior represents the alternative to experiencing oneself in some specific way—as some particular thing—that is so wretched as to be rebuffed by any means possible. If the celebrity parents mentioned above could bear themselves as people with normal children, they wouldn't be required to behave so unethically. If Pam could bear herself as a person who is not always unambiguously pleasing to superiors, she wouldn't be required to treat Kim so badly.

Thus, moral improvement requires one to relinquish something in which one is deeply invested in being. This is a pursuit that should not be taken lightly. It might sound like a simple task when read from this page, but as far as I can tell, it is in fact the unlikeliest of human outcomes. Think of it like this: even these celebrity parents, who live more comfortably than nearly 100% of all humans who have ever lived, are ready to risk jail time and public humiliation as a means of retaining "self as superlative." Think of the power it holds over them. They are enslaved by it (in our natural state, all of us might well be enslaved by something).

In this light, all maltreatment grows from an unwillingness to bear all one is, which is a problem of self-rejection despite that it often masquerades as a problem of self-regard. For example, many might conclude that these celebrity parents are moved by arrogance and grandiosity, that being "too taken" with themselves is their central defect. But why are celebrities ascribed grandiosity so quickly? Why would this kind of person be more prone to self-inflation than self-hate?[1]

Because expensive cars fill their driveways? One who thinks this way is in jeopardy themselves of being too taken with money and material. Even if they can put on a more convincing (and expensive) charade so it appears otherwise, celebrities are no less prone to anything human than any other human, including the proneness of humans to hoard certain aspects of themselves and repudiate others. Incidentally, just look at the epidemic of celebrity suicides and ask yourself if "really great possessions!" are a viable path to self-regard or an antidote to self-loathing. This is a philosophy that could only emerge in the fever dream known as the modern world, where nothing is valued like material is valued.

The Irresistible Mind: Identity, Come-Hither

From this perspective, the course of immoral behavior begins with simple identity. Whether conscious to us or not, when we are the maltreater (and all of us are sometimes) we are gripped by some version of the process laid out below.

TABLE 9.1 Identity and its Vicissitudes

Phenomenon	Real-World Example
When people invest in limited experiences of self, there are fewer and fewer modes of being that can be experienced as acceptable.	Someone who is only acceptable to themselves when they are "superlative" will experience negative emotion and deficiency when the external world challenges their experience of self as superlative.
Experiencing oneself as "X" is ideal because it results in value for the self.	He or she will strive for specialness in their pursuit (and maybe attainment) of "celebrity." Ideally, they will be perceived as special by all.

People come to be "not X" for reasons related to normative life processes that are unavoidable.	He or she has a child with a non-celebratory IQ, causing the superlativeness-bent parent negative emotion (e.g., embarrassment and sadness).
Despite emergence of "not X," "X" must be retained.	To retain their needed experience of self (i.e., self as special), the celebrity buys their child admission to top colleges so they [and their child] can still be superlative.

The great irony here is that at the very point one is unethically grasping at the only version of themselves they can tolerate (X), it has already dissipated; in fact, the very fact of its disappearance has catalyzed the maltreatment. For example, Pam's maltreatment of Kim is meant to push back against an unwanted self (*self as disappointing to authority*) and retain the wanted self (*self as fully respected by superiors*); however, this very act—the maltreatment—serves precisely as the indicator that the former has already appeared on the scene. In fact, she is responding to it. Her preferred experience of self is already out of reach. Were it not, there would be no need to chase it down, ever so destructively.

From this lens, ill-treatment of other people is done in the name of an unfettered yet unconscious illusion. Were the maltreater to verbalize the goings-on of the intrinsic world that precede harmful behavior, it would be said like this: "I cannot *yet* bear myself as that-ness (self as Y), even though *I am* that-ness; I can only bear myself as this-ness (self as X), so I must use others to push that-ness away." The person doling out the maltreatment, however, *cannot* put the process in such terms because, to them, all they *believe* they aren't, they aren't. But they are wrong. Too allegiant to their minds, they believe the content of their cognition determines who and what they are; in taking their identity to be derivable through thought, they truly cannot know that their self might be comprised of things that they *don't think* it is (let alone, *can't think* at all). For them, the self is what they consciously take it to be; therefore, upholding whichever version of the self they take themselves to be, at any and every cost, can only ever mean to that person, the *upholding of truth*. In this misunderstanding, they appoint themselves the grounds to treat others poorly, for in their attempts to retain self as they (consciously) know it, they always feel they are acting on behalf of something valid. In reality, they are beholden to illusion: the *non-self*, whose emergence they fear, however troubling, is so too *self*.

Only when a person can lose themselves (i.e., lose the self they prefer)—*and still tolerate themselves*—can he or she be good. Can't tolerate a self with normal kids? You might bribe colleges. Can't tolerate a self that is not admired? You might mistreat coworkers. When life is properly characterized as the impending mismatch between that in which we are invested in being (i.e., our current of experience) and that which we actually are (i.e., the ocean of experience), all immoral behavior shares one simple purpose: it aims to overcome the essential reality of shifting experiences of self. Each of us has different experiences of self we would prefer to keep at bay, but the moment we use other people as pawns to push them away, we are acting unethically and unrealistically: we have forgotten that reality so too includes *this*. Nothing is *that*. That-ness exists only in concepts. In experience, there exists only *this-ness*.

For anyone who really grips this model of poor conduct, it poses a genuine moral quandary. The experiences of self in which we have invested *can never be*, at least not completely or permanently, yet we mistreat each other thanks to our illusion that they can. Short-circuiting maltreatment, then, is accepting every aspect of one's experiential self, period. This would obviate the need to treat others as tools since there would exist no experience of self that our own comfort needs require us to reject. From this view, a great moral burden lies before anyone whose eyes are open: maltreatment, while unethical, also protects us from those selves we fear and hate, which means we have a choice to make. We can be safe or we can be good—but we can't be both.

The Modern World: A Petri Dish for Illusion and Suffering

Unfortunately, a quick survey of the contemporary world reveals that it has succumbed, probably irreparably so, to values that celebrate perfected and permanent selves, both of which are magnificent illusions. One place this pathological notion manifests is social media, where people appear bent on deceiving others—but more importantly, themselves—into all kinds of myths about human life. Whether pains are taken to advertise infinite beauty, importance, or charity, internet personas present to the world a fantasy of that which people would be if they could be, but are not—*at least not exclusively*. Even those aiming to rebel against social media norms by presenting a more mundane and realistic view of themselves have fallen into the same trap. Consider Instagram posts or blogs that are curated precisely to undercut curation, and instead meant to show what "real life" is like—whether the mom showing the world how little glory there is in scraping together a Tuesday pot roast, or the fashion model with sufficient "irreverence" to take pictures of herself from dawn to dusk—gasp—*without makeup*! Both might claim to be exporting something like authenticity—a needed island of realism amid an ocean of falsity. They might even claim that their "brand" is authenticity; but this is an oxymoron, since peddling anything like it's a pair of sneakers is a form of marketing.

The fact is that technology allows people to advertise themselves (i.e., to their "followers" and themselves alike) as superlative in whichever respect would most inflate them; that is, *in* whichever sense would most reinforce the conception of themselves with which they most identify. Where morality is defined by the coming to terms with all that we are, the reader should be wondering if access to such technology, which fosters self-deceit by way of self-caricaturing, could mean the end of ethics. Of course, it could—and here is how.

More time spent constructing and advertising the self one most needs results not only in *less genuine appreciation*, but worse, *more genuine disdain*, for the real course of human existence, which is defined by loss. Whether our losses are located in the self (losing youth, health, or quick-wittedness); in the material world (moving from one house to another, picking up and leaving a beloved town); in our relational life (moving away from those we love, the death of people we love); or in a more psychological or spiritual domain (losing a feeling of zest or losing some capacity for tenderness after a horrific event), *we* are always losing something as it once was. For this reason, all our attempts to define the self, to convince ourselves of its permanence, or even its stability, must be misguided. These efforts are attempts at inoculation from the changing experiences of self that define our existences. Though utterly human, understanding oneself as an enduring quantity represents an ethical crisis of the highest conceivable order, for what will we do when life shows us our everchanging nature? Simply, we will take it as evidence that something has gone awry. But nothing has.

Between our incredible medicine, online fantasy lands, and utopian ideals, even the existentially aware could wonder in 2022 whether all of life's problems are an error—a kind of mutation that the just forces of modernity have momentarily overlooked but will soon extinguish, in order to generate the world's very first paradise. Our modern values, for all of their upside, create a devastating problem. What happens when someone becomes convinced deep in their heart that perhaps all the difficulties of life are alterable, that perhaps wanting something means deserving it, and that perhaps all discomfort, loss, and sorrow are gross impositions? From that outlook, any encounter with one's *real* limitations, *real* faults, *real* discomforts become intolerable. They are then treated like noise, like nuisance, when in fact, they are the headline: they are the very signal that one is *completely alive*.

This is the problem with treating our struggles as if they need to be destroyed. Our struggles make us. They give us life, and being alive is contending with them, readily, freely, even happily. When we see life in these terms—instead of somehow trying to engineer human experience to perfection, whether by Instagram, surgery, or Artificial Intelligence—we do something that no one can see: we bravely relinquish the experiences of self we most need, and we bravely welcome others. This, a pursuit *of* the human soul *by* the human soul, towers in nobility, significance, and utility over *every other end* we human beings could possibly seek—every other one.

The Overlooked Ethical Organizer: Sadness

The moment one sees that the truth of being *is* the chronic loss of self, he or she also sees strident efforts to retain it as non-sensical, both practically and morally. Modern man has come to believe that he is a worthy adversary of existence itself, that in a battle against existential truths, he might come out on top. He is wrong, though, and worse for it. His entire existence is aimed at retaining self as is, which is a way of keeping as opposed to losing; and, ultimately, a method of avoiding sadness. Unfortunately, the joke is on him—and those he cares about—because only when one is sad, only when one can see, accept, and experience the repeated losses of self that define human life, can one be good.

Otherwise, life becomes the staunch, righteous, and always unethical pursuit of an abiding self, the first casualty of which is basic human decency. No matter what experience of oneself one rejects, it is rejected because it promises consciousness new, novel, and unknown qualities. It assures change, which, assuming sufficiently developed sensitivity, assures at least some sadness. We only need to think about life for five minutes to see how avoidant of grief we humans are; but think all day and we still might not link our reluctance to grieve with our capacity for maltreatment. This is a grave and consequential error.

Unfortunately, modern man's capacity for real and true sadness, which can help him say goodbye to lost experiences of self and better navigate related flux more generally, is especially compromised. So many of his wishes have come true, he is very often agitated (or even put out), but only rarely saddened when an unwanted experience of self emerges. He has a terrible time with grief because it appears to him as a hurdle to be gotten over, not an ethical end in itself. For this misunderstanding, he will suffer assured moral failure. The following are two examples, found in my clinical work, that demonstrate the eternal relationship between *the refusal of grief* and the *maltreatment of others.*

The Overbearing (and grief rejecting) Mother

Instead of being sad that children grow up and the terms of parenting change, a mother who fancies herself well-intended sabotages her daughter's every attempt at individuation. She pays for "background checks" to be done on all of her new boyfriends; worries publicly about their faults, in order to advertise herself as a deeply concerned (and not controlling) mom; and she encourages her daughter to live at home since each new beau is suspect. Whether her daughter's new love interest has spent the last ten years in prison or in the clergy has no bearing on mom's behavior. In fact, we must see that her skepticism has nothing to do with the situation at hand. Despite the fact that she might not see it as such, the whole charade is an illusion that thwarts profound sadness: she is no longer the needed mom she once was. Who can fault her for being sad about this loss? Nobody can, but there is no world in which this relieves her from the burden of becoming ethical. The mother's path to morality, and to better treatment of her daughter, is marked by the relinquishment of experiences of herself that no longer exist, as opposed to the desperate, destructive clinging to a version of herself that has vanished. Instead of being a mother who is now needed less than she once was, she remains intrusive, involved, and mistrusting of her daughter's autonomy and competence, mistreating her daughter and her daughter's love interests in the process. *She cannot grieve* what she was, and so she mistreats (all the while feeling "protective" and "loyal").

The Immature (and grief rejecting) Husband

Instead of being sad that his marriage was once fresh, exciting, and highly physical, a husband finds a newer and younger woman because doing so allows him to experience himself—once more—as sexually vital. No humane person would see his wish to retain this version of himself as immoral. However, we must be realistic: it is a wish absent any respect for the experiential truths of long-term intimacy, which certainly include things like habituation, mundanity, and ennui (as well as many other extremely positive qualities). In lieu of bearing an updated version of himself that is less spry, vibrant, and desired, he pushes it away via sexual impropriety. That is, he refuses an experience of self for which he is not ready but is already here (approximately: "self as aging"). In order to not mistreat his family *again,* he will need to practice the voluntary acceptance of new, less desirable experiences of self. But if he is to do so, he will need to achieve a level of *legitimate sadness* that has thus far evaded him. *Until he can grieve what he was,* he is a potential threat to his wife and daughters.

My point here is to show that for problems like these, solutions do not exist in the external world. As for the intrusive mother, no technology can prevent children from growing up; and as for the unfaithful husband, no advancement can prevent people—men or women—from wishing youthfulness would return (at least from time to time). In both situations, the only solution is the growth of internal worlds.

Accepting Means Accepting All

Those in psychiatry and related fields can be heard claiming that self-acceptance is the bottom-most solution to human life—and we are right. Moreover, what I am offering in this chapter likely sounds like a version of it—and it is. But we as a field refuse to bear what acceptance of oneself actually implies. Ultimately, it is a loving and compassionate act; and because it is, we take it to mean acceptance of those things for which we unnecessarily and unrelentingly punish ourselves. This category of things can range from accidentally burning the lasagne, to gaining 15 pounds over the winter, to forgetting to congratulate our son for his good grades. Yes, self-acceptance certainly means cutting down on destructive and indulgent self-criticism. But so long as we are moral creatures—and we are—it must also mean something more.

If we want to accept the whole truth of ourselves, we must also accept into our identities that which we push away for less sympathetic reasons than our proneness to being "hard on ourselves." In this category are traits like malice, self-centeredness, vengeance, remorselessness, selfishness, pettiness, meanness, and hatred. Since the beginning of time, these traits have been easy to find as one group has always seemed, to everyone, disproportionately afflicted with them: others. Acceptance of oneself is the highest aim, but it includes more than facets of being for which we criticize ourselves and should not; it must also include the facets of being for which we do not criticize ourselves and should. Self-acceptance is only a remotely respectable pursuit when it includes both; and when it does, there is nothing more important or life changing. The real development of conscience changes behavior like little else can.

The Infinite Availability of Moral Change

This chapter was filled with examples of people harming other people. In every case, the bottom-most reason for injurious behavior was their reticence to come to terms with the qualities of self that have come to constitute subjective experience. The more intractable, rigid, and defined one's idea of themselves, the more intolerant one will be of shifting experiences of self (i.e., of reality). Whichever self we prefer, we will lose; whichever self we prefer, others will set in. Our intolerance for any of them results in a pressing need to preserve the self as one knows it. The self known as an unrepresentable mode of being, nor the one known as a conception of mind, will stay. Requiring either of them to persist is the very point at which other people become casualties in our story.

Along these lines, the worst of human behavior grows from a simple misconception: that one's ideas of what one most is dictate what one most is. As alluring as it might well be, this view is an inbuilt illusion of the mind. Because Pam *thinks of herself* as respected and powerful, she can't bear it when she isn't; because celebrities *think of themselves as special*, they can't bear it when experience shows them otherwise; and because an aging husband *thinks of himself as a vigor-filled beau*, he refuses that which his immediate experience presents to him—strong evidence to the contrary. No, what we think of ourselves does not have the final say in who we are. Nothing could be further from the truth. When a person fails to grip this, he or she will try treating the ocean of experience—the whole of which we are subjected to—as if it could be selected from like a brunch buffet, thereby bringing sure harm to those in their orbit.

If what I have offered in this chapter leads to a prescription, it is one to meet every new day filled with an insatiable longing not to regain *what was self* or to engineer *what will be self,* but rather, to wholeheartedly surrender to *what is self.* While this view mandates people to almost obscene bravery in the face of every experiential reality, it is nothing like a heartless view of people and their lives. To the contrary, there is a single outcome of seeing the good life as one that asks people to become fully prepared to enter into their own psyche, torch in hand, and willingly *set fire* to experiences of self that are no longer, no longer useful, or just no longer here, at least not right now; there is a single outcome of seeing the good life as one that requires the feverish relinquishing of all one has been, in favor of all one is. The single outcome is mercy. Nothing else makes any sense. Mercy must be even higher than courage if we accept that none of us can be so brave as to give up *that which was* in every instance doing so is necessary. Furthermore, if we cannot accept that even adaptation, another word for loss, is inherently painful for people, we might demand it of both ourselves and others too stridently, thereby coming too close to ruthlessness. For everyone, sometimes being anew is too tall an order, at least right now.

Moreover, moral improvement, which only emerges by accepting all one is, can be a harsh task, but it isn't harshness—not ever—that helps people to do so. Nobody, not a single person, accepts truth when packaged in something hard and unforgiving. In some ways, this is the whole secret of psychotherapy; and in my estimation, it is the cardinal ability of everyone I've ever known who is considered by those around them to be unusually skilled in helping other people. It is the ability to help people abandon those ways of being that are unethical, morally deficient, and corrupt, all while upholding a psychotherapeutic treatment that is not punitive, coercive, instructive, or righteous. This becomes rather easy to do when one sees clearly the real obstruction to improved conduct and more ethical living. The details of that which has led to harmful behavior will vary from person to person. However, there is something that will not vary. The ethically troubled person, more than every other kind of person, has not fully accepted into their experience of themselves all that they are. Their needed experience of self is the most intractable; it is all but necessary to them.

As such, the task of improvement also varies in its details but not in its essence. Such people must become more than what they currently are, whatever they currently are. There is always and eternally more to be. The real self, the one bounded and defined by experience itself, must grow; while the illusory self, the one thought-out by mechanisms of mind, must shrink. None of us is what we think we are. We are all much more than that. However, this is not something any of us can learn through reason nor force nor argumentation; we humans will learn such a lesson only through something much closer to love.

Note

1 Incidentally, these phenomena always turn out to be two sides of the same coin.

10

THE CONTIGUITY OF BEING

All effective psychotherapies share something. Whatever the patient's "DSM diagnosis," the therapist's "theoretical orientation," or the theories either might use to explain change after the fact, all known psychotherapeutic "mechanisms" converge into one essential phenomenon. In fact, if life is becoming easier for a person at all, whether by way of psychotherapy, having found God, or having finally found work, the same process is being satisfied. The current chapter is my attempt to describe this process, for which much groundwork has now been laid. I will do so by offering a model that, in accounting for the fundamental, inbuilt problems of being, serves also to point at its solution. This discussion will clarify the essential mechanism, at least as I see it, behind not only all useful therapeutic encounters but all human healing—all things restorative.

The Contiguity of Being: A Primer

In any given moment, unwanted experiences of self might emerge; and even when they haven't, they are always as near as the next blink of our eyes. Thus, hardwired into experience are identity threats—threats to the non-conceptual *experience of self* we know, (i.e., we "are"), threats that take the form of newly emerging *experiences of self* we don't know (i.e., we "aren't"). As a means of keeping ourselves free of the suffering that would accompany new experiences of ourselves, we push them away, yielding psychopathology in general (Chapter 8) and injury to others as well (Chapter 9). As examples, our star employee from chapter eight, so resistant to experiencing herself as valuable, suddenly develops symptoms of depression in the face of a promotion. Or consider Pam, from last chapter, who treats Kim with outright malice in order to push away an already emerging yet unwanted experience of herself (i.e., self as unpleasing to authority).

DOI: 10.4324/9781003305286-14

Symptoms and immoral behavior ward off not that which reality is calling us to be, but that which reality has already made us.

We, unfortunately, refuse to be things, despite being everything—and *this* is the fundamental root of human harm. It doesn't exist in the pages of the DSM, in the case conceptualization a colleague presents, or even in the words I am using to describe it. It exists exclusively in experience, in being itself; it can only be apprehended there. Pursuing it in any other form is to pursue a ghost. In fact, our ability to know about and talk about these identity threats give us the false sense that we might also right them with cognition. But we have been fooled. In doing all of this, we are only playing with concepts, whereas the phenomenon *itself* never exists in our thoughts, our books, or our mouths, as it *itself* is not something to be represented. It *itself* is only something to be lived. One can already see that *the realest* sympathy for human beings must be aimed at the being part of it. All of us are being, and that's the hard part, whichever human we happen to be.

This perspective holds that being does not become full of pain, hurt, and misery through things having gone wrong, which is a very modern and shallow idea. Rather, by its very nature, the structure of being guarantees such things. It might well be true that certain brands of human suffering are explicitly worse than others, and that the worst kind of suffering is tied up with the worst circumstances. However, experience itself, *the being of existence*, is the native source of human suffering, even if the *circumstances of existence* pile onto it (which they surely can). Thus, the model presented here aims itself at working out that problem, the one we all share completely, even if we share nothing, visibly. It might also help us understand the most shocking, abhorrent, startling problems the world has ever contained, by helping us understand the deepest ones it has ever contained: those contained in you and me, the very deepest, most harmful, most chaos-producing of which is our simple but natural reticence to let consciousness expand when it is called to do so.

The philosophical aim of the model is to de-pedestal thought from the sacred position it has acquired in our fully taxonomized, modern world. An irony here needs mentioning. The model I put forth below is not free of the same language-based systemization it aims to deemphasize. This is a fact. However, it aims not only to *take into account* those features of life that are opaque to language but to elevate them as the most important part of human experience—and therefore, of therapy. The model assumes and admits that models are a failure.

Finally, the model is a response to so-called therapy brand names (e.g., cognitive behavioral therapy [CBT] *vs.* psychoanalytic), which draw the field's attention much more than they should. As a field, we have the problem of assuming that the *only thing* going on in a therapy room is the *thing we are aiming to do*. The cognitivist believes their patients improve thanks to cognitive restructuring; to the behaviorist, gains are produced by environmental manipulation; and for the psychoanalyst, the unconscious becomes conscious, thereby clarifying previously unknown motivations. The illusions of power and competence built into these viewpoints are astounding, but that's not the point; the point is that regardless of the verbally elaborated paradigm to which we adhere and set out to enact in the therapy room, there exist phenomena over which we have no power and which we cannot observe. There is always something else going on. To refuse this is to claim perceptual omniscience. There is an intrinsic world underneath words. If psychotherapy is going right, it is going right because of that which is happening here. This model would never claim to capture this world as concepts are unqualified to do so, only to point the reader in its direction.

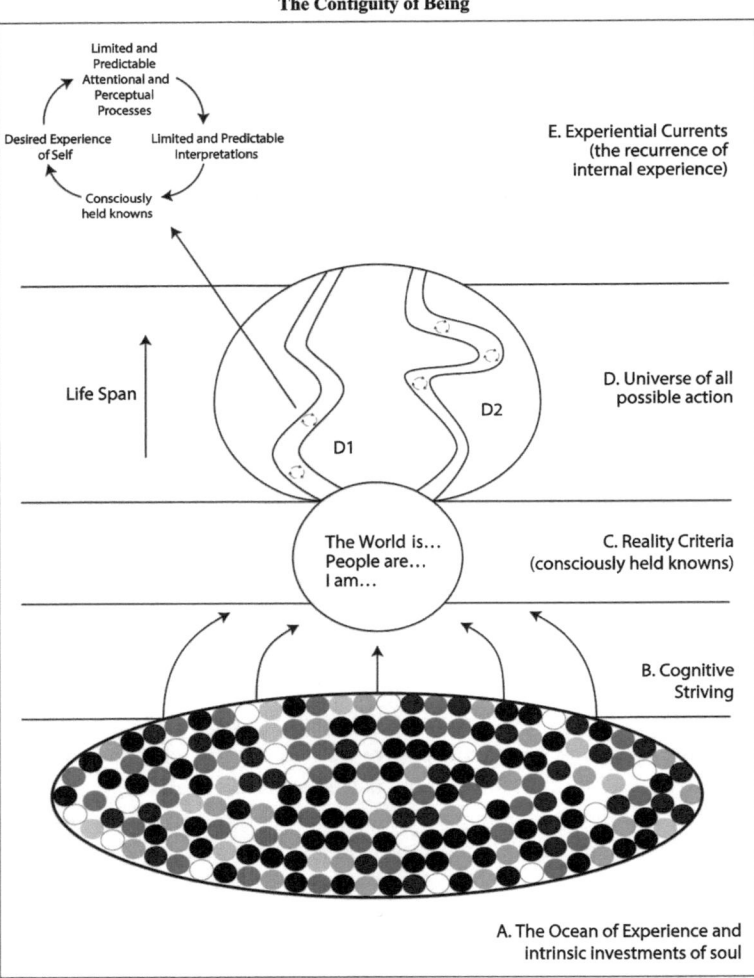

The Contiguity of Being

FIGURE 10.1 The contiguity of being

A Detailed Description of the Model

The Title

The model's name, "The Contiguity of Being," refers to its primary assumption: that "experiences of self" in which one is invested (e.g., in language, "being cold"), exist adjacent to those experiences of self in which one is not (e.g., in language, "being warm"), since one was unwittingly "chosen" *as the alternative* to the other, amid love interactions. As such, while new modes of being can seem infinitely out of reach with respect to time (e.g., imagine someone who has only known themselves as "hostile" for 50 years), as the intrinsic world of being goes, they are somehow within reach.

Part A: The Ocean of Experience and Intrinsic Investments of Soul

The large oval is a depiction of the intrinsic world, the entire ocean of experience, which envelops the total range of human subjectivity. All possible experiences of self are contained within the oval. The individual circles, differentially shaded, represent each possible experiential state that can be had by human beings, some of which we have labels for (e.g., self as "competent"), others we don't. The relative shade of a given circle (ranging from white to black) signifies the extent to which an individual has become invested in being *that thing* or experiencing the self in *that way*. Certain experiences are invested in completely (i.e., black circles), others not at all (i.e., white circles), and still others partially so (i.e., various shades of gray). Thus, the larger oval represents the parameters of the experiential ocean, while the pattern of shading within the oval represents the outcome of the cognition-free, investing process that determines what a person can comfortably *be*.

The following three points need to be made with respect to Part A of the diagram. First, the relative pattern of shading varies across individuals (the depiction above represents the state of one person's investments). More white space means that person maintains *less* capacity for being (it means a more limited, needed, and intractable self), whereas more black space means that person maintains *more* capacity for being (it means the self is freer to vary).

Second, taken together, all that is shaded within Part A represents one's experiential repertoire (i.e., what one *can* be), insofar as the gradation within each small circle (white to black) depicts one's relative comfort with the embodiment of that particular self. Related, if you isolated the completely black circles and ignored everything else, you would be left with that person's most common experiential current, whereas doing the same with completely white circles would leave you with those aspects of the ocean which remain untraveled and inaccessible to that person. Thus, the shading captures a person's likely, recurrent, and ordinary experiences of *this-ness*.

Thirdly and most importantly, the experiential this-ness produced by one's investments (i.e., by one's pattern of shading) *is* each person's deepest assumption, *is* the assumption on which all their mind processes rest (the one we failed to find *in cognition* in Chapter 2). It is alongside this nonverbal assumption that all mind processes take place; however, even calling it an assumption is to mix substances since it is not *known to mind*. More accurately, it is the unsayable quality permanently attached to our observation, perception, and interpretation, only to be found within subjectivity, that can never be said; it is the informulable apparatus (e.g., attention, perception, interpretation) through which all our consciously held formulations have been unavoidably run. It is *this-ness*, which can never be uttered or thought, from which all of our conceptualizations start and through which all of our conceptualizations must pass. This, a quality of consciousness that is not construct nor representation is our most consequential "assumption" and sits at the base of all we consciously hold in mind and "know."

Part B: The Striving Mind

The arrows in Part B of the diagram represent the trajectories of our minds, including both the unconscious and conscious processes that move them in certain directions (and not others). Cognitive striving is our mind moving along a particular path, heading toward particular conceptualizations and formulations (and not others); namely, those that are consonant with the experiences of self with which we are most familiar and comfortable. From one's experience of this-ness, produced by one's investments, all of one's cognitive activity grows. Minds, including how they attend, perceive, and interpret (i.e., how they strive), are beholden to this non-verbal "assumption." It might be said that while this-ness is not something we can represent, it is the thing *with which* we attend, perceive, think, and ultimately represent. This means that the way a person's mind thinks, interprets, and ultimately knows—the way it moves altogether—is a consequence of the experience of self fueling it.

As an easy example, a person who can only experience herself as "loyal" (and rarely if ever scrutinizing or skeptical or critical), is mandated to unnuanced ideas about complicated things. For example, she might proudly "hate" an admissions committee that decided to reject her best friend's application. Are there explanations for her friend's trouble, other than a dreadfully sinful admissions committee? Obviously, yes; but she has no access to them because her first principle, the first "assumption" from which her mind operates, is the *this-ness* that we would (in words) call "self as loyal." This quality of consciousness effectively truncates her own attention, thinking, and interpreting. In the truest sense, she cannot see anything else, but not because there is nothing else there. There is just nothing else there for her—for her mind.

People with very limited experiences of self are often the most certain of their minds for this very reason. They *actually* cannot see a given situation any other way because their mind is largely immobile (i.e., it can only move in a tiny number of ways). This is limitation. A bounded mind is the signature of an intractable self and a surefire precursor to not just vast misperception but grave ethical shortcomings. For example, unbeknownst to the loyalist, her ethical "system" is fated to become defined by the *abandonment of actual* ethics, as the judgments and interpretations her mind turns out will be necessarily limited. Without fail, they will be dictated by the actor involved, and *never* the act that took place—all because her cognition both works from and is meant to engender a necessary experience of self: "self as loyal."

Part C: Reality Criteria

If Part B represents the movement of a mind (i.e., the path toward its eventual formulations), Part C represents where it lands (its resultant formulations). Part C depicts the mind's thinkable, verbalizable products. Reality criteria are the places to which our striving minds have delivered us, places that take the form of concepts, necessarily. Reality criteria consist of every conclusion on which one has consciously landed and assumes to maintain a reasonable truth probability. All one would say is true—all the concepts and conceptualizations one endorses, along with all the ways they fit together or don't, represent one's reality criteria. The key here is that all one *consciously* conceptualizes as *so* (i.e., reality criteria) is intimately tied with what one "knows" oneself to be, non-conceptually, in being itself; it is intimately tied with this-ness which has emerged from one's investments (i.e., from Part A). Thus, the experiential state that one experiences as self, though it can never be thought or said, creates the parameters, boundaries, and outer limits of all one can think or say.

Here, we also see that despite our conscious view of things, our minds are, at best, secondarily motivated by a sense of accuracy, and primarily motivated by a sense of self, a sense of this-ness that doesn't *mean self* (which is too cognitive and therefore removed), but that simply *is self*. By way of the conscious realities one's mind derives from the external world (i.e., reality criteria), one manages to fortify their most comforting experience of self when it is present, and to retrieve it when it is lost. Think of the man on the train (Chapter 8). At risk of losing his needed experience of self (in words: "specialness"), he becomes briefly psychotic and deeply worried that his fellow train-goers might even be *too* interested in him. His mind moved in such a way that the self he experiences as *most him* was spared. This is what minds are after. This is the nature of the safety on behalf of which minds work (discussed in Chapter 3).

Here we see that while the formulations on which people have landed can be argued about, debated, and evaluated in and by the galaxy of thought, they are attributable—ultimately—to something not to be found in thought, something that cannot be thought. Our mind processes, which we believe are adherent to the external world, in the deepest conceivable sense, are *adherent to* and *maintaining of* a needed experience of self, a "thing" without representation in mind and without verbal correlates (even though I can couch it in words, time after time, as the experiential "this-ness" that has emerged from one's investments in specific "experiences of self").

Part D: Universe of All Possible Action

Part D of the figure above is meant to depict the observable paths of two differ- ent lives (D1 and D2). These paths are a consequence of both people acting on behalf of their respective reality criteria (i.e., knowing what the world *is* lends one to *corresponding* action). Since differing action emerges, at bottom, from differing investments, it should be noted that these hypothetical people would also main- tain different patterns of shading in Part A.

For one person, their reality criteria (i.e., *the world* is a task; *people* are meant to work; *I am* responsible) might ignite conscious goals to become educated, get mar- ried, raise kids, work 70 hours per week, and leave little time for leisure. Another person's reality criteria (i.e., *the world* is enjoyment; *people are* meant to experience comfort; *I am* flexible) might spark concerted efforts to find warm and affiliative relationships, work that isn't too taxing, and pursuits always containing some pleasure.

Their different formulations of reality account for their differently shaped lives (depicted in the path of D1 versus the path of D2). They will do different things, meet different people, and find themselves in different places. In other words, there *really are* visible, undeniable differences in how people live, which *really are* attributable to what people consciously know of reality (as discussed in Chapter 4). Thus, despite having arrived at them for reasons we cannot say, our conscious knowns—our reality criteria—are hardly irrelevant to the trip of life. In the beha- vioral sense of it, captured by Part D, knowing different things yields very different lives. However, while lives can look as different as different can be from the out- side, they are in one sense the same—all of them. All lives, all *interior lives*, are bound by recurrence.

Part E: Experiential Currents (the recurrence of internal experience)

Part E of Figure 10.1 is meant to more thoroughly represent the currents of internal experience that emerge from one's investments in self. They are depicted multiple times along *the same life path* (e.g., D1) in order to signify that they are naturally prone to recur, independent of a person's circumstance (i.e., indepen- dent of time or place); they are depicted *across life paths* (e.g., both D1 and D2) to show that they are always operating for everyone, even if the content contained in them varies from person to person (which it does); and they are depicted as cycles in order to indicate their repetitive nature. The key point is that, for everyone, internal experience recurs. Let me now detail the cycle, which is meant to be read from left to right, using a case example.

E1: The Desired Experience of Self

One's desired experience of self (i.e., desired state of "this-ness") follows from the nature of their investments in the intrinsic world of being, which were made in love. Let's take a young, career driven financial expert as an example, and let's assume that the *experience of himself* in which he has become invested would be characterized (in words) as "self as dominating." Remember that while we can put words to this investment, as we just did, it doesn't operate as a concept in experience but as a mode of being that he finds desirable.

One can imagine many early experiences to which he would have intrinsically responded (i.e., without the help of cognition), by investing in this mode. Perhaps his love objects (i.e., Mom and Dad) were hapless and helpless, unable to provide him any sense of security—emotionally, financially or otherwise. Thus, he would have received no love that wasn't a bit compromised—all of it was incompetent, inadequate, and ineffectual. Since it *provided him nothing usable, actionable, or worthwhile,* if love is to go unharmed—if love is to be spared—it must be something from which he needs nothing. He therefore invests in those experiences of self that will make being—that will make him—precisely needless (e.g., self as strong, hyper-competent, and dominating). Had he invested in the opposite experiences of self (e.g., self as reliant, unsure, and less than competent), the love he received could never have been good enough. Thanks to the former set of investments, love has never been inadequate or caused him suffering; what's more, were he to invest into these experiences with enough force, he might avoid suffering altogether. He might be impossible to harm (which might be the whole point).

E2: Limited Attentional and Perceptual Processes

At any point along his life path, his attention and perception will have the same goal: to produce—or at least not disrupt—the experience of himself he so needs. This is the way in which people are exactly the same, regardless of whatever distinctions simple observation uncovers (e.g., cultural background, wealth, day-to-day circumstances). While the experiential quality (i.e., the this-ness) that people are after certainly varies, the fact of being after it does not. Whether he is in the boardroom, at the beach with his wife, or at his 40th high school reunion (place); and whether he is in graduate school, mid-career, or retired (time), his mind and all of its processes strive to yield the experience of self with which he is most comfortable. The happenings of the actual, external world, whatever they *actually* consist of, become mere fodder for the production of the desired experience of self. The world is attended to and seen in such a way that his bottom-most assumption, the non-language-housed experience of self he so needs, is retained when present and restored when absent.

E3: Limited Interpretive Processes

The pool of interpretations and conceptualizations he is capable of realizing is only so large, since the movement of his conceptualizing apparatus is constricted, given that it is shaped (co-opted) by the experience of self in which he is invested (which, in moment-to-moment life, amounts to this-ness). The quality of this-ness that constitutes his experience (and follows from an investment in "self as dominating") drives his attentional, perceptual, and, ultimately, interpretive processes. Importantly, his interpretive apparatus—and its properties that move it down one track and not another—can never be verbally delineated, since they are not made of language, exist exclusively in experience, and therefore refuse to be tracked with concepts. That is, his interpretive apparatus can only *do*; it can never be *said* (even if we can refer to it as this-ness or anything else).

However, we can see what *all of its doing* yields, thereby seeing something of its spirit. Of our finance friend, we might know that while watching a professional baseball game with coworkers from the firm, he is more likely to interpret the players as "idiotic gorillas" than "modern day gladiators with divine skill." The reason for this is simple: if he viewed them in the latter terms, their potential for dominance in the world would threaten his. His preferred experience of self would be jeopardized. Thus, his interpretations are limited by his own investments—and the stronger they are, the more pruned and truncated his interpretive apparatus.

E4: Reinforcement of Reality Criteria/Consciously Held Knowns

From someone's *Limited Interpretive Processes* (E3), come their *Consciously Held Knowns*: all one consciously takes as true (i.e., their reality criteria). From the baseball game mentioned above, our finance friend might take as real the proposition: "athletes are morons." He *knows this*—as opposed to something else—because it is more likely to engender the experience of self he needs (i.e., self as dominating). This idea was also shown in Chapter 5 (via Harry): reality criteria are not easy to impeach from within, nor are they are coincidental. They give rise precisely to one's preferred experience of self. This is also why, in Figure 10.1, consciously held knowns (E4) are depicted as *feeding into* one's desired experience of self (E1). It isn't merely that one's preferred experience of self fosters their reality criteria; it's that their reality criteria fosters their preferred experience of self. For example, with his conscious view of the athletes (E4), our young financial expert is back to E1 (i.e., the experience of "self as dominating"), and the cycle starts over.

On Contiguousness: Past is Present, Present is Past

From this perspective, in any given moment, a person's being repertoire—what one can and cannot be—is determined by their *then operating* pattern of investments (i.e., their idiosyncratic pattern of shading in the intrinsic world). This pattern could be thought of as the sum consequence of all past interactions, and more particularly, as one's response to the nature of love constituted in them. This begins to mean that a person's history is always internal to them, never behind them.

This is not a philosophical point but a practical one with real implications for the moments we spend with patients. It means that to be respectful of a person in the here-and-now is to be respectful of the whole of their past; that understanding what a person can and cannot be with you, *in this moment*, is to understand what they could and could not be with precious others who came before you *in past moments*; and perhaps most importantly, that helping a person to be in new ways with you—in the here-and-now—is to work directly on their history, whether it seems obvious or not to those who take the world as one populated by discrete events, disconnected from each other by the concept of time.

Time surely passes; but it is only our minds that equate passing time with permanent changes in our experiential repertoires, whether positive (e.g., being less sad) or negative (e.g., being more callous). In the *intrinsic* world—that is, in *the realest world*, which cannot be conceptualized—experiences of self are not in the past, nor are they in the present. They merely are. The intrinsic world is populated by every possible experience of self—all different, all available, and most importantly, *all contiguous with each other*.

When a person really understands the contiguity of being—the landscape of invested-in and rejected experiences of self that occupies the intrinsic world—they understand that regardless of when, how, or why our ways of being were established, different ways of being so too exist, despite their apparent absence. What's more, *this-ness*, subjectivity as any of us experiences it, has resulted not just from those experiences of self in which we have invested (shaded circles from Figure 10.1) but from those in which we have not (white circles from Figure 10.1): it is the hodgepodge of our investments—the *pattern* of shading in Part A of Figure 10.1, which includes all its constitutional elements, shaded and not—that has made subjectivity into *this*. That is, it is our relationship with the *totality* of the intrinsic world that yields this-ness (subjectivity as *this*). When consciousness as we currently know it (as we currently experience it) is the aggregation of *all of our* relationships with *all of our* potential experiences of self, something rather strange is implied. We must be in perpetual contact not only with those aspects of human experience that, despite existing, we are not currently invested in being; we must also be in perpetual contact with every aspect of human experience that has ever existed in all human beings that have ever been. Somehow, whether we seem to be or not, we are *always and eternally* connected to the whole of the ocean (whose potentials and limits are perfectly equivalent across human beings). This is the case regardless of what exactly subjectivity is like *right now*, since, whatever it's like, every element of the ocean—every circle, shaded or not—has contributed to it (i.e., to this-ness).

Past is Present: A Brief Case Example

Years ago, a patient (whom I adored completely despite her completely reckless hostility) marched into my office and sat down with such force that she cracked the arm of her (my) chair. She then says, "I need to use your computer. Somebody is getting fucking fired." I say, "anybody I know?" She says, "not unless you know the piece of shit cabdriver who just told me to smile because nobody died today. First of all, how does he know nobody died? Maybe my mom did, he doesn't know." I say, "So you're calling him?" She says, "No Rob, I'm calling his fucking boss. I didn't ask for his number after he verbally assaulted me" (she is very hostile and very hilarious).

I say, cheekily, "Lucky for him." She says, as angrily as you can possibly imagine, "Do you think this is fucking funny?" I say, "Not at all. I think it's serious—for you and him. He's gonna get fired and you're gonna have to deal with that guilt you always feel after you retaliate—you know, the guilt you feel even if the retaliation is totally warranted, which, if I may, I'm not so sure about here." She says, "Yeah well he didn't tell you to smile." I say, "I guess that's true. But one time, years ago, I did stay on the phone for six hours straight, just to get a customer service rep fired. He made the mistake of telling me that he thought he'd never say so, but I, the customer, was completely wrong. I think he also made the grave error of calling me completely stupid."

Ava then cracks a smile. She did not expect a self-disclosure and frankly neither did I (the number of times I have, unprompted, offered something about myself to a patient are all but nonexistent[1]). But she was especially surprised by this one, wherein I look so perfectly unhinged. After all, there I was, sitting across from her in a sweater and docksiders. She certainly didn't know 23-year-old me, but they would have been fast friends—so I introduced her. For the next 40 minutes, we laughed at how absurd people can be, including me and her, when they feel offended—and how unnecessarily destructive. We then started to wonder what her cabdriver's story was. We asked what might have happened to him on that day that made him so preposterously bitter. He did, after all, insult someone for no good reason. The plots we created were ridiculous, hilarious, and mostly unrealistic. But they were so enormously helpful. By the time she left, she wasn't looking to have anyone fired (or killed).

Many "responsible, scientist-practitioners" might describe this session as a nonsession, marked by a lack of direction and a lack of adherence to stated goals and all-important treatment plans. My view of this perspective is that it is (almost) irreparably inhumane and outrightly stifling to the human spirit. That session had *everything* to do with the treatment plan: help Ava become less miserable. It also had everything to do with her history. How so? Because we were *being light-hearted* together instead of *being punitively hostile*, the latter of which was an experience of self chronically available to Ava; on this day, however, she was able *to be* the former.

Over time, sessions like this helped her release an intractable self by which she was constantly gripped. In this particular session, we spent the entire 45 minutes being collaboratively outrageous (not an intervention you will find in any textbook), which helped her to "laugh off" an impulse to destroy a stranger, which would only have further damaged her already damaged soul. Moreover, in creating hypotheses about the cabdriver's motives, though many were purposefully absurd, we managed to wonder about him, his mind, and his experience, which is an essential part of developing a peaceful interpersonal stance. We have to see how others see; at the very least, we have to be willing to wonder how others see. Without this, a path to peace isn't one.

On that day, were we talking about the cabdriver Ava encountered 10 minutes earlier, in present-day, adult life? Sure, explicitly, we were. But we were also talking about whatever—whomever—it was in Ava's life that first compelled her to an insatiable thirst for blood and vengeance when forgiveness would have better served her soul. This was not a behavioral intervention intended to impact her "supervisor-calling behavior," as it would be described in a behavioral treatment plan. It was an intervention into the meaning of things like punishment, retribution, aggression, all of which had a hold on her that she was always powerless to fight—at least by herself.

Our preferred modes of being, though developed by way of the past, are situated in the present, within us; and therefore, carried around from one moment in time, one point in space, to the next. The manner in which these modes interact with the real and actual external world *is the history* operating in the now. Thus, while past and present are separate entities in our minds, as the world of being goes, it begins to seem that they are somehow united, forever inseparable. And this is true. *That which is* can never be parsed from *that which was*.

As time goes for Ava, *the funeral at 40* isn't *her brother's hockey game at 19* isn't *the family picnic incident at 16* isn't *the kitchen table at age 11* isn't *the living room when she was seven* isn't *the vacation to Florida when she was five* isn't *the car ride home from the hospital.* But it also is. They also are the same. Because of the contiguity of being, they are also each other: our intrinsic response to any given event (which takes the form of an investment that produces particular shading in Part A of Figure 10.1) maintains both a permitting and constraining function—i.e., a determining function—over our available range of future responses, since it delimits via diminishment that into which we *can* invest. Simply, every moment represents, without exception, the unfolding of prior moments. This means that a person's history is encounterable, purely, perfectly, and without dilution of any kind, in every passing moment—if we only look for it. As for the question raised long ago in the Preface—"does the past matter to the present or does it not?" This is a bad question. The past is present, always.

The Model's Implications for Psychotherapy: Dethroning Thought

This model is meant to cast one's desired experience of self, which is not accessible with mind, as the key obstruction to updating, editing, or revising what one *knows* in one's mind. To the extent that we humans aim to reproduce the experience of self to which we have grown accustom, and we do naturally, we can *never* know the world anew. To some inescapable degree, human cognition is aimed at keeping intact (when it is present) or generating (when it is absent) the subjective experience—*the this-ness*—with which we are most comfortable. This is why minds misconstrue and misconstrue.

For example, does the finance guy from above really believe athletes are primitive gorillas? In one sense, yes. But in another sense, we don't really know what he thinks because as things currently stand, his intrinsic need for superiority and domination is driving the bus of his thought (recall E1 through E4). If he were suddenly able to *be more* than just these things, his mind's attentional, perceptual, cognitive, and interpretive processes would look quite different. They would become freer. More technically, his conceptualizing apparatus would become freer because that which drives it, which cannot be conceptualized (i.e., the experience of self that has grown from his intrinsic investments), would be expanding. In turn, he would land on and incorporate novel ideas, attributions, and formulations. He would develop *new knowns*.

Thought Does not Move Thought

This model thus undermines most contemporary psychotherapy protocols, which concern themselves with two components of the diagram above. They are first concerned with Part B, insofar as they aim to change how people's minds move (i.e., the "think like this, not like that" essence of cognitive restructuring); and thereby, they are concerned with Part C insofar as they aim to change where people's minds land (i.e., a conscious "take" on reality that is more consonant with reason and evidence). Basically, cognitive therapy aims to explicitly reroute the striving that goes on in Part B of the diagram above, with the goal of altering the consequential contents of Part C (i.e., what one arrives at as *true* by way of cognitive striving).

Such a treatment might endeavor to teach someone to think in a different direction with respect to other people, themselves, or even their own thoughts and feelings (an intervention into B), the purpose of which would be to alter the conclusions they consciously draw (altering the reality criteria of Part C). For example, after a dose of CBT gone right, our paranoid patient from Chapter 7, convinced that the cashier hates him, might enter a grocery store more equipped to think his way to the conclusion "people are not terribly interested in me or what I buy," thereby allowing him to receive the gaze of the cashier—and others—in innocuous terms. In turn, he could see them in the same way, and shop more peacefully.

While changing what the patient consciously knows (e.g., about the people at a supermarket) is an excellent goal, the cognitive approach to doing so rests on a faulty assumption: that a person has *chosen* how their mind will strive. If someone had really thought their way to their way of thinking, if they had *deliberately* decided to think how they do, then helping them to *deliberate* further about the manner in which they think might turn the tides. It would help them to see the (literal) error of their ways—and presto!—they would decide to utilize superior patterns of thought. This perspective, modern life's favorite intervention for helping people, represents a near-total misunderstanding of human beings.

A person who has never quite been able to see themselves, others, and the world differently; never quite been able to see or think in new ways; never quite been able to adopt a new "attitude" or "mindset" defined by new and better conscious knowns, has not fallen short of such changes because other ways of thinking are *inaccessible* to him. He has fallen short of such changes because other ways of thinking are not viable to him. To see this, recall Harry. He has considered all the evidence for the possibility that his friends very much appreciate him—he has even *thought* they do. What he cannot do is believe in that thought because doing so would not fit with the experience of self in which he is invested (self as undeserving), the one that drives his conceptualizations and interpretations of the world. For a short period of time, such a thought might freely sit about the banks of his cognition, contemplating itself, weighing its viability; but eventually, it will be picked up, incorporated, and swept away by the entrenched rush of his cognition, which is beholden, finally, to the experience of self propelling it. One can think what they want, but if those thoughts are not consonant with the investments one has made in who they are, they will first be empty, then overpowered.

From this view, not only is thinking not the *source* of maladaptive thinking; stranger still, nor can it be the *antidote*, since it does not contain within itself the resources to alter itself. Cognitive therapies aiming to instantiate and make viable *new* cognitive behavior using appeals to one's cognition *as it now stands* are engaged in a fool's errand: what they see as the apparent tool (the patient's conscious thought) is beholden to the actual problem (the patient's intrinsic investments that drive it). Imagine coming across a shattered hammer in the road and being told you must fix it, but you are only allowed *that hammer* to fix it. This is the nature of expecting thought, as it currently stands, to make itself anew. Neither the impediment nor the bridge to new conscious thought exists in conscious thought. Both exist in that which moves conscious thought: the unconceptualizable, intrinsic investments that rule with an iron fist the movements of one's mind.

That Which Most Moves Thought Cannot Be Thought nor Touched with Thought

This next problem turns out to be a problem for every therapeutic modality, not just cognitive approaches—not to mention, every practitioner. All theoretical orientations, whether CBT, psychoanalytic, or anything else, invoke a conceptual frame for making sense of the other's thinking. After deciding it strives how it does, thanks to "automatic beliefs" (CBT) or "internal conflict" (psychoanalysis) or anything else, every theoretical orientation then invokes analogous tools for helping a patient to revamp their thinking. At bottom, these tools take the form of words. We know this because therapeutic conversations are deemed relatively "psychoanalytic," "mentalization-based," or even "integrative," as a matter of the language that constitutes them. Whatever our theoretical orientation, we implicitly expect the therapeutic interactions most fitted to our theory's concepts to hold the most power to help the patient revise their cognition (i.e., to help them arrive at new conceptualizations, formulations, and interpretations—new reality criteria—about the world).

None of this sounds too unreasonable until we see the claim it amounts to, in terms of Figure 10.1. Whatever its pet objective (e.g., unearthing conflict, restructuring cognition), we are claiming that the right kind of interactive speech—*the right kind of dialogue*—can not only puncture and gain entry to Part B of the diagram (where the patient's mind *actually carries out* conceptualization) but also tweak that which is idiosyncratic therein (i.e., that which causes it to move how it currently does), thereby redirecting it, so that it finds its way to new formulations (so that "C" becomes populated with new propositions—new knowns).

But how could language do this? Everything said by both patient and therapist is *itself* a conceptualization. The entire conversation therefore takes place in Part C of the diagram, unavoidably so, meaning we have overshot our target entirely, assuming we meant to intervene into the inputs of conceptualization, thereby changing its outputs. In opening our mouths, in having something to say whatsoever, we have only outputs. The conceptualization ship has already sailed. Thus, words alone cannot "tune up" the most idiosyncratic feature of one's conceptualizing apparatus, the one that causes one's mind to strive toward the conceptualizations it does, not only because this feature is made from this-ness, not words, and therefore cannot be tracked or touched with words; but moreover, because all the words one could speak were *made from it*. And so, if we have used language at all, we have already utilized and left behind Part B, since the *doing of conceptualization* that takes place there—and which refuses verbal or cognitive capture—*has brought into being* the formulations and conceptualizations (i.e., propositions) we and the patient are now speaking.

In thinking about what moves thought, whether on our own or with a patient, we have never found what we seek. Every time we think we are holding in mind that which moves thought, we are first holding that to which thought has been moved. Therefore, getting "a verbal hold" of how and why we think how we do, as a means of changing it, is much harder than it seems, arguably impossible. Here is an interesting parallel. If while walking down the street, a stranger asked you for directions to the train, you would probably provide them with an explanation. A few blocks later, if you saw a beautiful bird, you might shout, "Look, a blue jay!" Both cases, the *explanation* provided to the stranger and the *declaration* about the bird, represent the *products* of mind. Nobody would ever think twice about this. Yet, somehow, *explanations* and *declarations* as to how one has come to see and think about the world as they do, when stated in a therapist's office, are assumed to represent the *causes* or *antecedents* of mind.

However, the act of thinking or saying what has caused us to attend, perceive, and think as we do, can only ever be an expression of our attention, perception, and thought *as it now stands*—even if we label it in words a "cause" of these processes. There is nothing we can think or say that is not beholden to the manner in which our mind *now is*. Therefore, nothing we can say is a cause of how our mind works, even if we label it one. It's just our mind working; it's just an expression or an effect of how our mind *now works*. As a result, conscious reality criteria can be said (e.g., I take "X" to be true of the world), but what has gone *into* them, what has *made* them, cannot—not even by exceptionally educated, well-intended, highly intelligent clinicians.

Real Transformation

Thus, one of our field's major assumptions might be off base. Psychotherapy is meant to explain and intervene into the way someone's mind works. However, if someone's mind has come to work how it does via processes that cannot be conceptualized, then products of further conceptualization (i.e., co-created hypotheses, insights, and explanations) simply fail to explain the "thing" they are aiming to, for this very thing resists explanation. We assume that in helping people develop more conscious theories about themselves, we are giving them the tools to alter *how they attend, what they see, and what they* think; but we aren't because these same tools can never penetrate the place *from which* they attend, see, and think (i.e., the investments in self *with which* they do all of the above).

Fortunately, in seeing this error, we also see a more viable path to genuinely revising what one knows, what one holds in mind as true (i.e., one's reality criteria). A better approach would be to alter that which one's mind is intrinsically aimed at, via altering the quality of consciousness—the experience of this-ness—forever attached to its manner of perceiving, thinking, and interpreting. Crucially, this can only happen *at the level of intrinsic investments* (Part A in Figure 10.1). Changes there would lead to a mind that departs from a different quality of experience and therefore strives differently, thereby finding new formulations and conceptualizations (Part C). If we are serious about "restructuring" thought in a remotely meaningful or lasting way, we need a tool for "restructuring" *the intrinsic*, which is not thought and cannot be thought but somehow actuates and directs thought.

Cognitively Based Protocols: What's Really Happening?

It needs to be acknowledged that protocols and didactically based treatments help people. I want to offer an explanation as to why, which will not be found in the psychological literature. Imagine a man who has become chronically homicidal after discovering that his wife has been having an affair. His hostility is so palpable that his employers, his kids, and even his poker buddies (a quite rough crew) agree that he is behaving worse than his wife ever did. Over several weeks of an "anger management protocol," his aggression dissipates to manageable levels. The treatment plan involved presenting to him new information (in the form of new skills), through which he learned to reroute his murderous lines of thought (a cognitive intervention), reduce his physiological activation (a physiological intervention), and rearrange his day in order to encounter fewer hate-producing stimuli (a behavioral intervention).

Remember that the whole treatment dialogue consisted of conscious conceptualizations—his and his therapist's—meaning it took place entirely in Part C of the diagram above. Nonetheless, it *really did* seem to change the movements and destinations of his mind. He stopped seeing his wife as evil, he stopped thinking his way to images that induced rage, and he became increasingly prosocial. These are good outcomes. The question is, how did such interventions, which aimed to rewire conscious thinking *at the level of conscious thinking*, help him? Well, they didn't. Throughout treatment, something was going *on at the level of Part A* (Figure 10.1), despite that every word, every concept, every protocol-rooted suggestion, was utterly powerless to get underneath Part C.

Thought processes marked by less hostility and murderousness only open themselves to people invested in *being peaceful;* streams of attention lured by the tenderness in the world, not the barbarity, shine forth only for those invested in *being gentle;* and a perceptual gaze imbued with forgiveness will only materialize for those invested in *being merciful.* Thus, knowledge transfer, attempts at using propositional language to replace "maladaptive" lines of thought, currents of experience, and perceptual paths with "adaptive" versions of each, *can* in fact work—but not for the reasons we think. If knowledge transferring approaches have worked, they have fostered a shift in the investments a patient has made in who they are—even if unintentionally (as is often the case with preordained "protocols" through which thought technicians attack all of the "symptomatology" that populates the construct world). Even when therapy is aimed in a decidedly scientistic direction, the therapeutic action is the same: something has been touched in the intrinsic world, in the world of the patient's investments.

Yes, our angry husband learned how to complete a "thought chart," but he also learned that he might *be someone* whose own thoughts matter enough to be attended to; yes, he learned how to ward off self-destructive physiological activation, but he also learned that he might *be someone* who ought to handle himself—and his fury—with more care; yes, he learned techniques to replace seething resentment with gratitude, but he also learned that he might *be someone* for whom overcoming hatred is worthwhile; yes, he learned to structure his day so as to avoid "anger-inducing stimuli," but he also learned that he might *be someone* worthy of cultivating peace. Throughout the entire treatment protocol, all the while his mind was being treated as if *what it thinks might not be so accurate*, he was being treated, ever so simply, as if *he might be more*. The latter—not the former—is how his thought, and eventually his behavior, changed. His intrinsic investments, which once limited his mind to certain movements, had now grown, thereby affording it much more mobility.

Psychic Progress is an Avalanche of Investments

Let's now remember that a person's pattern of investments in the intrinsic world (Part A of Figure 10.1) is a "quantity" permanently unknown to cognition—both theirs and ours. The substance of which it is made cannot be put in terms of mind. If this goes unrecognized, we become too pleased with our ability to "know" how a person needs to change. Shortly after that, we assign ourselves the role of master chef (i.e., you need a dash more of this trait and a touch less of that one). This approach defines knowing someone in the wrong way because it follows from our needs (a way of relating to another that, at its extreme, arguably defines evil). If we believe a person should "stop being that way and start being this way," it is only a matter of time until force is applied to reach that end. This is one problem with knowing too much: eventually, it gives way to a pressuring orientation. It makes clinicians more rule-bound and strait-laced, and less creative and free.

What's worse, in setting out to force divestment from Trait X and investment in Trait Y, we are not being true to the ocean. People are everything. Whatever we take people to be in our minds and fantasize about changing—e.g., their pessimism, haughtiness, or vapidity—is a trait that, like all traits, is first human and only secondarily "problematic" (an overused and divisive fixture of modern parlance). As a result, picking them as if they are weeds—aiming to help people *divest* from certain experiences of self—is the wrong tack. The right tack is to grow more around them—to grow *that which is contiguous with them*. This is the work of investment. It is aimed at growing, not shrinking; embracing, not shunning. It is aimed at life, not death. We humans are not recipes to be perfected nor weeds to be picked; we are dormant selves to be awakened, uncultivated selves to be grown. It is the expansion of investments that constitutes all human healing, all things restorative. And so, we therapists want to set off an avalanche of this very kind: *more* and *more* and *more* investments in what one is, gaining *more* and *more* and *more* speed, until one can freely experience themselves as everything they are—as everything the ocean of experience is, always has been, and always will be, eternally.

The best psychotherapeutic method, then, is one capable of growing the other's investments, no matter how they now stand, a "standing" unknowable with mind. But is there a method for the general expansion of the other's consciousness, period, no matter its current state? Or do we have formulas exclusively for moving the other's consciousness in the direction we think it should be moved, as determined by cognition's manner of representing it? These questions are to ask how one person might help another person to invest in all they might be, regardless of what they now are, the latter of which cannot be known by mind.

This brings us to possibly the strangest thing about helping people and the constitutive tenet of being useful to another; it is also the thing most refused by psychotherapy protocols that first medicalize people, then "fix" them. It goes like this: one person can never truly show another person that alternative ways of being are acceptable. This is an ontological impossibility because alternative ways of being can never exist in the here-and-now. And if they come to exist, they are no longer alternative; they are in operation. This acknowledgment puts us clinicians in an odd situation. Our goal is to help another person grow into new, previously unembodied modes of being, but all we ever have to work with is the way of being that is, the way of being that is operating right here and right now—however we might label it, whatever we might think about it. In turn, the question for therapists becomes, "how would we interact with another's current mode of being in such a way that new modes of being are fostered?" The answer to this is very easy to say, very difficult to do, and opens one's eyes to see the very heart of psychotherapy.

In response to whichever mode of being a patient happens to embody right now, we treat it the same way: as well as we possibly can. Helping someone to be *more,* and graciously embracing them in the way they *happen to now be,* are only different things in words. As the being world is concerned, they are eternally, unambiguously, and unequivocally indistinguishable. They are one. The simplest yet deepest truth of psychotherapy is that people get better not as their variable experiences of self are more and more loved, but as *this one is.* Our field is threatened by this idea—and rightfully so because it is so unspeakably powerful in its simplicity that it threatens business as usual, the business of "getting to work on people," "doing things for them," and changing them with sanctioned versions of "force, expertise, and teaching."

We must be good to people. As compared to being smart and competent to people, being good to them wins. It wins all day, every time. Why? Because being treated with goodness is what affords people the most opportunity to invest in more experiences of self, which is the essential condition of all human healing, all things restorative. So, what is being good to someone? It can be many things, but each of them follows from first *going with* them.

Note

1 I would also note that this was the only time I told her anything about me, which is why it stands out now. Somehow, I was just responding, and a self-disclosure exited my mouth.

11

COMPASSIONATELY GOING WITH:

Psychotherapy is a Dance on the Brink

I hope the reader has gleaned from the text thus far, especially chapter ten, that while thought and language are psychotherapy's most manifest currencies, they couldn't possibly be its deepest. This is not to make cognition into a clinical shortcoming; after all, every therapeutic encounter is defined by listening, thinking, and talking—by dialogue. What's more, if observed by a fly on the wall, some of the most valuable therapy sessions would be summed up as two people "thinking together," albeit in a distinct, even peculiar way. Such encounters are marked by engagement, an often messy "joining together," the key characteristic of which is the wholly felt freedom of both participants. There is an implicit agreement that both people are, first, free to verbalize *any and all* thoughts; and second, free to do whatever they want with what the other offers—whether that be revise it, reject it, ponder it for one minute or the next 44, immediately incorporate it, mock it, or anything else. Psychotherapy, when done right, looks like two people who have silently agreed that their minds will be absolutely unrestrained together. At its best, a therapeutic encounter is an experience of being completely awake and alive *with another*. It's two minds dancing.

Still, the actual dialogue of dialogical exchange can never *be* experience; it can only represent experience. In terms of Figure 10.1 (in Chapter 10), *no conversation* takes place within Part A or B, even if every one of its constitutive verbalizations has its roots in both. This is because Parts A and B contain processes that *both* cannot be said (or thought or cognitively tracked) and contribute to whatever is said (i.e., a conversation's emergent content). While the entire text of a conversation belongs in Part C of the diagram (as Part C houses the finished products of conceptualization, representation, and "propositionalization"), language nor thought can ever capture the experiential core from which these processes (and their final products) grow. This core is confined to first-person experience, never

DOI: 10.4324/9781003305286-15

to exit it on the back of words. Thus, the best dialogue can be is *about* subjective experience.

Yet nobody has ever walked into an intake session with a new therapist and claimed that their problem is "*about* subjective experience," or that they hope psychotherapy helps them speak and think differently "*about* subjective experience." But nor are they merely trying to tell us of some problem that is *in* subjective experience. What they want us to know, the meaning of which cannot be conveyed with words alone, is that their problem *is* subjective experience.

Remember that human suffering exists forever in subjectivity—in the intrinsic world—as the struggle to be a certain way, thanks to heartfelt investments in being another way. This is a drama that takes place not in cognition, even if it can be depicted there, but forever in being. Human harm *is* too few investments in what being *really is*; put differently, it is the existence of outstanding swaths of ocean yet to be invested in and made self. Its solution is incorporating more *this-ness*, more consciousness that genuinely *is* self.

What Can and Can't be Represented: A Brief Review and Implications

Throughout this book, I've been referring to intrinsic investments with adjectives (e.g., self as needless). Before moving forward, it is essential to reemphasize that such words do not squarely map subjectivity. Here is an example. If 100 people observed Ned for a week and agreed that he is "domineering," this characterization would still say nothing of the subjective state of *being Ned*—this state cannot *be said* since conception and language can only represent being. This disparity is perhaps clearest when people use their thought in order to represent themselves. For example, imagine Ned fully agreeing that he is interpersonally troubled by his manner of "dominance." That is, *being dominant* is a problem for him and he knows it. Why doesn't it help Ned to "know" this? Put differently, if he can represent his dominance and name it as a problem, or at least a source of unneeded tension, why doesn't he just stop being it? My answer to this question will sound irreverent and cheeky, but it isn't intended to be, so please take it seriously: for the same reason he couldn't stop his house from burning down by aptly *characterizing* it as "on fire" and representing on a piece of loose-leaf paper every chemical interaction that has produced it, is now sustaining it, and will eventually extinguish it.

It isn't that our characterizations of experience are valid, only futile to help, but rather, that they are valid in terms of the world that created them: the world of thought. This is not to say that a boastful, know-it-all like Ned is "wrong" to characterize himself as "arrogant and domineering." He isn't *wrong* exactly. It's just that "arrogance" is a signifier, and thus, a signifier *of* something else. But of what? For this chapter, I want the reader to imagine the ocean of experience (Part A from last chapter's figure) as an ocean of phenomenal states, as the simple felt-ness of being that cannot be represented (as opposed to the adjectives by which it can). In this light, one's pattern of investments (represented by idiosyncratic shading) would not yield a descriptor, a combination of descriptors, or some theoretical average of descriptors. It would yield something truly confined to experience, never to be found in cognition.

Over the course of this book, I have termed this indescribable experience, *this-ness*—it's just subjectivity as *this*. But verbally elaborating what I am referring to even as "this-ness" *is* to represent it *is* to alter it. In other domains, we easily see this disparity inherent in representation. This is precisely why, when it comes to a fire, we call a firefighter armed with a hose, not a chemist armed with a periodic table of elements—because we want to alter "it," not "it as elaborated by sophisticated verbal representation." In therapy, patients can tell us with words who they are and who they aren't. They can offer us "causes" and "antecedents" regarding how their minds came to work how they do. They can tell us more than they have ever told anyone. All of these can be facets of great therapeutic encounters. Yet, all of it takes place in the world of representation—the construct world. Despite that this information can tell us how patients represent their experience, no such activity can deliver us to the aspect of first-person experience that makes it *theirs*. Nothing thought nor said can be a bridge to the way a person experiences themselves—to the inexpressible *this-ness* that has been produced by their intrinsic investments. When we think it can be, we misconstrue both the meaning and target of compassion.

Psychotherapy, Concepts, and Compassion

In all it does, in all it assumes, modern psychotherapy takes *experience as represented* to reflect *actual experience*. "What's depression?" It's this list of symptoms. "What's PTSD?" It's that list of symptoms. "What's the treatment for this kind of anxiety?" It's that sequence of maneuvers. This view of human life is simplistic and silly, but worse, it jeopardizes our field's relationship with compassion.

When a listener hears a speaker describing their experience and conflates it with the speaker's actual experience, something strange happens: words become much too important. Eventually, the speaker's verbal representation of experience will somehow be heard as the speaker's experience itself. At that point, what else could earn the listener's compassion but the speaker's manner of conveying—of representing and verbalizing—what they are experiencing. In such a scenario, it isn't subjective experience but the concepts by which subjective experience is portrayed that come to matter and mean to the listener. And by what metric will the listener assign importance to the speaker's concepts? Well, by the extent to which he or she identifies with those same concepts, of course! But assuming we are therapists (not cheerleaders) and listening (not rooting), this must not be the right way to hear people. It's only a good way to agree with them (when attached to the same concepts they are) and disagree with them (when not).

However, all of us, not just therapists, have to make judgments about what other people say, including its rightness versus wrongness, truth versus falsity, and wisdom versus foolishness. There is no way around this. No meeting of minds is absent such evaluations because all minds naturally assess whether other minds make any sense to them—and eventually, they won't. This is true of every speaker-listener dyad, which is defined by two separate minds. Luckily, compassion is not necessarily lost each time patient and therapist conceive of the world differently (i.e., hold different concepts about it); but when compassion is lost, it is often for this reason. A clash of ideas or perspectives—of concepts—often yields conflict, or at least something less than compassionate understanding.

This truth confuses modern psychology, though, which has concluded in response that the abandonment of cognitive judgments must be the clearest path to a compassionate interpersonal approach. The rationale goes like this: if one isn't making judgments, no concept to which the patient is attached will be criticized or thought poorly of, and in turn, interpersonal harmony will abound. However, even if they have done so with good intention, those who have ferociously judged non-judgment to be an achievable standard for human beings, are naïve. Our field needs to address this bunch. Instead of accounting for the mind's defining process—discernment—they brush over it, pretending it isn't there. But it is there. They often learn so when they are finally forced to admit that this or that patient's conceptual scheme—whether conservat*ism*, liberal*ism*, femin*ism*, environmental*ism*, traditional*ism*, or anything else—has made them so upset that they can hardly sit in the same room as the person who has sought them out for help.

It would help all of us to understand judgment not as a moral failing but as a cognitive fixture. A person who has *truly* eradicated judgement would wake up, hear their alarm clock, and not know whether they should turn it off or fry it for breakfast. If one has successfully given up discernment as a practice, expect them to be laying in a heap wherever they happened to first manage it. After all, they would have no hierarchy of "next moves" if evaluation itself had been properly exiled from their mind. And so, if someone is functioning in the world—if they are dressing themselves, going to work, and eating enough so they don't starve—and *also claiming* to have overcome their mind's judging apparatus, they are ruled either by self-deception or naivete (first cousins). For therapists, neither is an especially welcome trait. People don't call us because we appreciate fairytales, but because we appreciate reality.

My point here is to expose a nonsensical philosophy. Our minds are tools for judgment and scrutinization. We can all be honest about this. In fact, it's so clear that it shouldn't even require honesty; after all, we don't muster honesty to say that fried eggs beat out fried alarm clocks, do we? Even those who erroneously take their minds as naturally non-discerning can surely imagine "unnatural" situations in which judging would feel quite right—perhaps even invigorating?

There are certain things—thoughts, feelings, and behavior—that each human will feel compelled not only to judge but to criticize and condemn. No person in good faith can claim to have given up judgments because there is no mind that isn't perpetually making them, including the minds of terribly refined, enlightened (often performative) psychologists.

To solve the problem of judgment, some therapists convince themselves that while acting as therapist, the high goal is to work extra hard in order to breed non-judgment in *this setting,* within *these* four walls. But this is foolish. It is akin to reducing the likelihood of getting into an accident in one's new car by removing its engine. The trouble is not only built right in; the trouble is what makes it go. So long as a car is a car, there will be risk; so long as a mind is a mind, there will be judgement. Of course, mine is no argument for open criticism of other people. It is anything *but that.* Rather, it is to show that if we really want to accept people, we might well need another vehicle; cognition, overvalued in the modern world, will not get us there.

Compassion that runs on and allocates itself as a matter of the ingredients and contents that comprise the other's mind will soon run into a brick wall; compassion that dispenses itself as function of the acceptability of *the other's concepts*—their reality criteria—will be short-lived (not to mention false for the whole of its lifespan). This kind of compassion will soon be withdrawn, and to the extent that the person supplying it misunderstands minds—and they do, necessarily—doing so will feel justified and right. But it never is. No two minds have adopted the same concepts, the same reality criteria, and no two minds are supposed to. For a higher kind of compassion, one that makes *no requirement* that the other identify with the same conceptual reality criteria we do, thought must be de-pedestaled. For this kind of compassion, the conscious mind is a broken vehicle. By its nature, it is permanently flawed. No matter how smart, kind, or well-intended one is, the world of cognition—thought—is an ever-crumbling bridge to the other.

So is not true of the *intrinsic world*, the only world people will surely find one another. Every experience of self *that is*, is shared; yet no experience of self is a cognitive representation. This view clears the brush to a truer compassion, especially when it is shrouded in conceptual and ideational gobbledygook. Having trouble mustering compassion for someone with whom your refined mind disagrees? For someone whose behavior makes you bristle? For someone whose conscious political views are reprehensible to you "and anyone decent?" For someone who represents the world 180 degrees differently than you? Then, I have good news: there is still something you share with them, something so profound that you'll never not share it. Can't find it? Stop searching your mind for "agreed on propositions" or "shared conceptions of reality." Stop searching your mind altogether. Instead, find the experience of self—the *this-ness*—that is currently gripping the other, *from which all of their conceptualizations grow*, and let it grip you. Find it within yourself. And if it's not there? Ah, then you've been fooled: it is there.

The Impossible Complexity of This-ness

I have used this-ness as a term that defines the quality of a person's default, ordinary subjective experience, which was produced by the intrinsic investments that one made (e.g., in being X or Y) amid early love relationships. But to more fully grasp the meaning of clinical work, this notion must be complexified. The investing process that creates subjective experience as one knows it—this-ness as one experiences it—does so iteratively and continuously. We chronically invest in what being will be, in what we will be, as a matter of our *ongoing participation* in the world. This phenomenon is in tension with but no less real than the phenomenon by which each person's being repertoire is somewhat established and baselined through their earliest, most consequential love relationships. The self, defined as a landscape of invested in and rejected phenomenal states, is somehow *both* set and indeterminate, not one or the other.

Thus, while the manner in which a person is *now* invested in being (i.e., their current pattern of shading from Figure 10.1) could be neatly conceptualized as "the outcome of all previous moments and the unwitting investments made therein," subjectivity doesn't really have "outcomes"—not in real-time. So long as one is alive, one's current investments (e.g., in being X or Y) are perpetually subject to the same process that made them. Because each moment holds potential to impact those experiences of self in which one *is* and *is not* invested, one brings to each subsequent moment, each next interaction, at least potentially, an updated pattern of investments.

This means that at every point in time, each person has—*each person is*—a potential for being that interacts with (and might be remade by) the goings-on of the world around them. Depending on the nature of *this moment*, the self might be made anew by the primordial investing process—and anew, and anew. This is the case for every moment and means that the self—the one made via unwitting, intrinsic investments and experienced consciously as this-ness—is never static. Nor would it be amenable to plain verbal capture even if it was an expressable substance, not only because language somehow gives us both too much and too little to say about it, but because the investing process that defines it is ever-happening, ever-operating, so long as we are alive.

The self, then, can never be pinned down with words, which are useful precisely because they simplify: they make *stationary* and *treat like a finished product* that which, in fact, is susceptible to revision in this and every moment. Imagine driving down the highway and trying to state your exact geographic coordinates. The moment you open your mouth, the thing you are trying to capture changes into something else. This would be a more accurate way to conceive of the intrinsic self, the one that despite being parameterized by early experience, is also subject, somehow, to unqualified change. Technically, we might describe the self as an "ever-changing algorithm of investments, always in flux and always fluctuating as a matter of the invisible interaction between one's pattern of investments as they now stand (reflected in Figure 10.1, Part A) and the external world with which one is *now* engaging." But said more soulfully, we'd just say that, "yes, people are what they are; but in response to the relative love around them, they can expand in ways that transcend any conception of self that their mind, as it now stands, can conjure up."

The key here is to see that the self is much more like an *ongoing process* than a settled quantity. Because the investing process has no beginning or end—and instead just *is*—the self does not maintain distinctive epochs to be discerned, even if our minds, via delineating the self as a matter of time, can make them. This means that asking, for example, "why someone is X" or "when someone became Y" can only be done with any sense of viability, *whatsoever,* thanks to mis-understanding. This question freely attempts to apply the rules of one paradigm (the conceived of self) to a paradigm so different than it (the intrinsic self), that the person asking it is likely to be unaware of the latter. That is, their lack of self-awareness manifests in their assumption that cognition would be the best vehicle by which to become aware of the self. Anyone for whom *self* means *self as thought about* is not self-aware, not in the deepest sense. But this is common. People tend to see the conceived of self as primary when they take the primary feature of themselves to be thought; after all, the conceived of self is the only self available to thought. However, it is still secondary.

The self is not one thing, as concepts must be, nor can it be found in thought, as concepts must be. Thus, finding the *experience of self* currently operating in the other in its truest form as it now exists—as *this-ness*—must not be a job for cog-nition. First of all, there is a volume problem. The path of investments that has brought the self to this moment, that has made *this-ness*, is impossible to capture with thought because even if this path were delineable with cognition, there would be *too much* to think: imagine trying to grasp with cognition just exactly how every preceding *moment* of one's subjective experience had a hand in affecting their then existing investments, thereby bringing about the investments associated with the *very next moment*, and so on, until the whole sequence by which *these investments* populating *this moment* has been accounted for.

The second problem is more important and now more familiar to the reader: because the "investing process" takes place independent of thought, all the operations laid out in the first problem, those that define intrinsic changes to the self over time, are unthinkable. Thought can only tell a story about a changing self, but this story contains nothing immanent to the changes it underwent; even the truest narratives, as they have become observable via mind processes, must not con-tain anything of the untraceable investing process by which selves (non-conceptual ones) shift and change.

This can be quite hard pill to swallow, especially for those with a deep trust in their own mind to genuinely uncover the self, as opposed to merely represent and narrate it. Yet in its truest form, the self is some process that thought can never touch. For those who see the merits of this view, it means something as strange as it does burdensome. Thought is not the door to the experience of the other; even if we want it to be, even if we are very intelligent, even if we are very good at telling the developmental story of the other, thought cannot be the door to the other. It can only be a door to conceptualizing them. Really meeting the other is a test much too complicated for cognition—it fails every time. And so, the only viable entryway to the being of the other is through the door of being itself.

Toward the Other, not Conceptions Thereof

Imagine a very difficult patient—a young woman who consistently but unwittingly degrades every single person she mentions, except for those lucky enough to be either her blood relatives or her oldest friends. Per her report, and in defiance of all statistical probability, these groups are comprised of exclusively superlative people. Over time, our minds might tell us she has "narcissistic problems," "a superiority-inferiority conflict with all the trappings," or a "poorly individuated/differentiated self." In light of the discussion above, we can now see that however valid these characterizations might be with respect to the world of constructs, they move us no closer to her subjectivity.

Responding to our own conceptualizations about "how she is"—which are products of cognitive discernment and meant to carve up the world into "X" vs. "not X"—is to impose into the encounter a half-right distinction. While it is true that her mind moves differently than ours (Part B of Figure 10.1), therefore landing on different reality criteria (Part C) and causing her to take very different action in the world than we do (Part D), this is a truth to ignore (or at least to banish for a while). There is a deeper truth. The characteristics of her conscious mind and observable behavior, however different from the characteristics of ours, grow from something that could never be foreign to us, something to which we have eternal access: the intrinsic world of being. Because the ocean of experience is wholly shared, every region of it in which she has invested and *made self* is also right there, just waiting to be had *by us*.

So long as we have looked inward sufficiently, it is not possible to believe—it is inconceivable and *always* wrong to convince ourselves—that the experience of self currently sitting across from us, the one usually referred to as "other," is not also sitting within us. *Always*. In fact, when we go into the deepest recesses of the self, we find that there is no experience of self that is ours, nor is anyone else's experience of self theirs. Though both are observed as highly personal to the observer, they are not; here, observation fails. Every experience of self, every state of this-ness that seems unique to me or you, emerges from an ocean of experience that we share, entirely. As for the patient mentioned above, the deeper truth, which we want to somehow prioritize and make primary, is that if we stop thinking, we will find her lurking within us, won't we? We will find within *ourselves* every aspect of the ocean in which she has invested and made *herself*, won't we?

The rightful target of our attention, energy, and compassion must be the other's subjectivity since this is where suffering exists, but attempts to think ourselves there will fail. Thought keeps us on its fringes, never letting us puncture the subjectivity of the other, never letting us know it, not fully anyway, since we can only really know experience as experience, not conceptualization. We are thus left with a question: if we can never think our way to the experience of the other because the workings of mind can only further abstract it, thereby putting it further out of reach, what can we do? As alluded to back in chapter one, we must contact it. We must go with people, *into* experience.

On "Going With"

The Virtues of Not Knowing

"Going with" is to enter the experiential world of the patient by adopting the very intrinsic investments they have (e.g., self as X or Y). It is to understand this-ness in the only way it can be: not via conceptualization but from the inside, as a state of subjectivity. Not only does this pursuit not involve cognitive knowing; it is best achieved with an interpersonal posture of *not knowing*, which is orthogonal to a posture marked by concluding, deducing, and the like. But what exactly is this posture?

The suspension of knowing has to mean the suspension of verdict, of landing on this or that, or landing at all. It is to intentionally deprive oneself of "closure" (and all of its natural comforts, discussed throughout this volume). Inhibition of closure could be alternatively described as the cultivation of *doubt*. As language goes, doubt refers to something propositional: "I am not certain if proposition X is true." But let's leave this aside for a moment and ask what doubt means as a quality that finds us in experience, as a quality of being that populates us? It might be hard to say because we in modern life are allergic to doubt; or we think we are, and so we flee from it. In turn, we fail to understand its nature and the full reach of its experiential implications, and we rarely benefit from its virtue. If we can better understand the "in-experience" analogue to the concept of doubt, we can grasp why it turns out, paradoxically, to be a gift to those who have come to us looking precisely for final answers.

Going With: On Doubt

Everyone knows the saying, "don't mistake kindness for stupidity," but why do these things appear to go together in the first place? You might be thinking, "this doesn't mean anything, Rob; it's just some colloquial expression." Fair enough, but I want to discuss it precisely because it is so commonly perceived as to have earned its own expression. Somehow, clues that the other is *kind* overlap with clues that they *aren't so bright*. Whether or not it is true, empirically speaking, what is this connection about?

The first hint is to see the other side of the coin: people who portray themselves as being stocked to the brim with knowledge (i.e., "know-it-alls") are thought to be insecure or haughty, and are often disliked. But what is going on here? Does the possession of knowledge mean unkindness, whereas a lack of it means kindness? This would be odd. "One does not necessitate the other," says our cognitive assessment. Maybe not, but there is a reason they seem bound up together from within subjectivity. There is something real and true about this connection—and some part of us sniffs it out in the air of experience.

What we are really sensing is the signature of *foreclosure*. To the same part of us that senses someone as "knowing," they also register as "closed." Because knowing requires ruling out, it necessarily involves shutting down. In knowing, there must always be "closed-ness." One requires the other; thus, they occupy the same experiential air, necessarily. The knower's very posture sends a signal into the world around them that indicates a quality of fixed-ness. They read as someone who, insofar as they possess their own pre-validated answers, needs little from experience; in fact, the most severe knowers are people for whom experience has lost all its explanatory power. An individual like this could take or leave experience, and what they know—*what they believe they know*—goes unchanged. This posture of knowing, because it transmits foreclosure into the air between people, often creates a negative response in others. To understand why, we only need ask, to *what exactly* is the knower actually closed? The abstracted, out-of-experience answer is something like: "everything but their idiosyncratic knowledge." But the non-conceptual, in-experience answer is much simpler. For all of us, that answer is, "me." Happening upon "knowing" in another indicates, if only nonverbally, that the knower could so too, take or leave us. To *them*, the this-ness now populating *us* matters nothing. And somehow, we know it. How do we know it? We *feel* it, we *become* it, we are *touched by* it, we *sink into* it. Notice that none of this "knowing" is particularly cognitive in nature.

Now, we can see why dimness and kindness seem to present in the same experiential field. When we experience someone as knowing very little (i.e., being "dim"), we more readily experience them as "kind." What we are actually picking up on, however, is what their relationship with their knowledge means for *us*. If they are know-nothings, they could not possibly have foreclosed; and if they have not foreclosed, our experience could never be irrelevant, immaterial, or meaningless to them. They are, by the nature of their relationship with their "knowns," open—that is, open *to us*. We experience them, therefore, as having something approximating a kind posture.

The state of "not knowing," which in words is a reference to cognition, in experience, is an emotional tenor; specifically, one we might characterize as *tenderness*. Genuine doubt, as embodied via experience, not abstracted via cognition, is a quality of unmistakable receptivity. In real-time experience, not knowing shows itself in the simplest way, and however paradoxical, it means everything to someone who is seeking. Not knowing is a palpable openness of heart. It is openness of heart given by a power far beyond and utterly superior to cognition. Why is it so essential? Because it fosters finding the other in one's own being before one's own thought. As I will show below, this is precisely the catalyst by which the other finds themselves.

Going With: Know How is No How

Because "going with" is not achieved primarily with cognition, verbal instructions for carrying it out come up short, necessarily. In this sense, it is a process without a how, one that can never be said—only done. Were we to think of it as an act, it would be an exceedingly simple one. There is no volition in it; only a non-resistance to being swept away. There is no pushing in it; only an acceptance of being pulled. There is no doing in it; only a readiness to be done to. As it is an internal act, it maintains no discernable movements. It proceeds through the relinquishment of all destinations. And it finds what it looks for by abandoning the whole concept of a search.

Going with is permitting the consciousness of the other to wash over us, however it might. As it does so, we contact within ourselves the place from which the other is speaking, a place that is always accessible since all experiences of self are eternally shared. It isn't thought-fueled; it isn't imagining with our mind *how* the other's mind works; it isn't thinking about what it would be like to think how the other thinks. Rather, it is sharing with the other their location in the intrinsic world, the experience of self *from which* their mind is currently operating. Whatever the other is being—whatever being has become for them—we must *be it with them*. We must grip the experience of self now gripping the other; and to do so, we must surrender, completely and wholeheartedly, to being gripped by it. Importantly, this is a task internal to the clinician, and not necessarily observable; it isn't behaving outwardly in the way the patient is behaving, at least not necessarily. It's knowing the state in which the patient finds themselves by letting it emerge within oneself. It is knowing by way of joining, participating, sharing.

All the while patient and therapist are having a real and useful conversation, akin to the manifest "moves" of a card game, it is this underlying exchange that holds all the weight, the one wherein the therapist tracks the patient's whereabouts in the being world, and ever so simply, *remains with them*. This pursuit is totally unremoved from each moment, totally unabstracted, totally unmediated by thought, which means we cannot gain perspective on it. It never *happens*; rather, it only ever *has happened*. It doesn't emerge; rather, emergence is *it*. It is a process of which we can somehow be aware as it happens, but not "aware" in the cognitive sense. As it isn't a task of mind, some might hear this as a task of the body, others of the heart, others of the soul. Whatever its mechanism, I would only propose that this abiding capacity to contact each other, not through our minds but despite them—and despite *their differences*—be considered a gift from beyond.

Now recall our narcissistic patient from above, the one our mind has characterized in a largely negative way. Is there a way to respond to something deeper than our conceptions of her, which, let's be honest, include such notions as "thoughtlessly and unknowingly tyrannical," among others? There is. We must go to the place in ourselves that wishes for self-importance, for power, for specialness, for superiority—not that "once did" because we conquered childish dreams but that "once did, still does, and always will," since before anything else, we are the ocean, the whole cast of selves that comprise it—permanently, unavoidably, eternally. In rightly going with, it doesn't matter that we cannot in words delineate what her investments are (e.g., self as special vs. superlative vs. invulnerable), since they are palpable in the air between us, thereby allowing us to know them in real time, not in representation. They can be felt. They can be "be-d." We must welcome the experience of self that has become her by contacting it in ourselves. This is how we overcome the distancing instinct to conceptualize people. We let the qualities of *their consciousness* into our own by letting the properties of *their investments* become our own. Then, we talk with them from a shared place.

Going With: Because Intrinsic Investments are only Truly Alterable from Within

Finding in oneself the *experience of self* in which the other is currently invested has the effect of helping them to grow into adjacent, contiguous experiences of self, those in which they are not currently invested. In language, this amounts to the development of infinite multiplicities in the domain of being. We want someone to hold capacities to be both assertive *and* deferent, both joyful *and* despondent, both serious *and* silly. But we cannot aim directly at altering such thought-produced constructs. *Knowing* someone is "passive" (with a need for assertiveness) fails to be the first step in helping them transform in *exactly the same way* that knowing a raging fire is "fuel, oxygen, and heat" (with a need for buckets filled with twice as much hydrogen as oxygen) fails to spare your house. Just as a fire can only be put out by entering into it, contacting it, a person's intrinsic investments can only really be touched, not said, as they are not of the construct world; and thus, to alter them, they must somehow be entered into.

Speaking and thinking of the quality of subjectivity we want to change only couches it in cognition. It only cognizes it (it erroneously makes it an "it"). This tool can tell us about subjectivity, make great sense of it, and even conceptualize its development, but it can never puncture subjectivity itself. And so, the fire rages on. What we really want is to rearrange the other's intrinsic investments—to expand them. But as they are exclusively of experience—not conceptualization of experience—experience is the only true site of change. We thus must enter the fire. But we are still left with a question: how exactly does going with people into the experience of self *now gripping them* foster movement into *new experiences of self*? This is, after all, the whole point of psychotherapy.

Toward a Mechanism: The Action of Psychotherapy is Unavoidably Mystical

Being with someone in the *experience of self* now gripping them seems to remove the threat from nearby modes of being. It seems to extract the danger from the waters surrounding their current, which until now have been wholly inaccessible because of their promise to induce loss and loathing (Chapter 8). Sometimes abruptly, sometimes over long periods of time, people reinstate that which never felt missing—those experiences of self that despite having always inhabited the intrinsic world, have never inhabited them.

Recall Part A of Figure 10.1 (Chapter 10). Experiences of self that have been passed over (white circles) exist immediately next to experiences of self that have been taken aboard (black circles). Psychotherapy's so-called "mechanism" materializes on the brink between them—and the mechanism itself is *a bridge.* Where there was once only an abyss, emerges something solid that connects *this* experience of self, the one operating *right here,* with *that* experience of self, the one that has always been there, sometimes thought about, but never incorporated as self—never embodied.

What is essential to understand about this bridge is that it is not made of thought. Therapy's dialogue *does not* build the bridge; believing it does is to miss the real exchange for the card game. The bridge turns up not when the right words are spoken but when patient and therapist are genuinely sharing the same experience, and it turns up in the form of a simple sense. People willingly try on and invest in more aspects of themselves when they sense that the other's gaze has dissipated, when they sense no quality of division whatsoever—not internal to them, nor internal to us, nor between us and them. The bridge is made from a sense that there is *nothing other.* This makes it quite a bizarre bridge, since it is defined by the absence of that which defines normative, subjective experience and normative observation: a sense of separateness. In moments like these, every ingredient of internal limitation—which together mark the *very parameters* of one's default experiential current, the *very boundaries* of one's default being repertoire— suddenly give way. This fosters a strange *freedom to be,* and access to more ocean.

For all of us, our investments are naturally made, at least in part, from defensiveness; that is, we have come to be in the way that spares love, thereby keeping us secure. But when a person experiences the boundaries of their "currents," the limits of their "being repertoires," and the givenness and therefore the validity of "this-ness" as illusory, which they are, their primitive need to protect themselves is replaced with a more mature and exponentially more powerful need: the need for truth. The truth they are after, however, is not cognitive; it's not constructed. It is the deepest kind of truth. People want to know all they are, which is something different than all they think they are. That is, they want to *be* all they are. And so, they begin to explore all they are. They begin to traverse the ocean within. This is what *actually* happens in therapy, and it's *actually* imperceptible.

It consists of the patient and therapist venturing out and dabbling in new experiences of self, moving about the ocean, navigating it together, being in one state for a while, maybe a long while or maybe not, then moving out beyond that state to try on another, and so on. As the patient more freely contacts and spends time in the experiences of self in which they have not yet invested, they slowly *do* invest. For example, as one becomes more familiar with being assertive *in addition to* being passive, the two collapse into each other, which means one becomes fully capable of both. Their repertoire expands. In turn, one experience of self is no longer opted for—*desperately* opted for—over the other, as both are incorporated into one's being repertoire. What results over time is more control on the part of the experiencer: choice comes into the picture, as does *responsiveness to reality*. In a situation where passivity is best, passivity is embodied; in a setting where assertiveness is best, assertiveness is embodied.

Early in this volume I suggested that we need a vision of human improvement and psychic growth that applies to the intrinsic world, not the world of constructs. In terms of Figure 10.1 (in Chapter 10), relative progress *is* the gradual filling-in of every small circle, until there is no experience of self the patient has not made his or her own, and no experience of self that, if called for by reality itself, cannot be readily embodied. In terms of actual being itself, relative progress is simply one's felt expansion of consciousness, one's own experience of a growing being repertoire. What results from these changes is a person fully capable of confronting the external world and being in the world in the way they see fit. In being more and being more with more freedom, one is afforded agency. One develops a profound willingness to call on whichever experience of self is called for.

Important too, we human beings can never be in total control of ourselves. This is a grandiose idea; the ocean is a ride and, ultimately, we are not its operator. This is to say that certain situations will simply induce in us particular experiences of self. Crucially, once one has invested in all they are, even those experiences of self that do not feel volitionally chosen pose little threat. Peace with the tension defined by one's *power* and one's *lack of power* over the contents, qualities, and vagaries of subjectivity creates a profound ability to "go with the flow" of the ocean within. Amid such self-possession, life looks like all possible experiences of self freely coming and going, populating us then leaving, and bringing with them not only little bother but much delight, for this—and this and this—is also us, and so it should be permitted, tended to, and nurtured.

All psychotherapy is a dance on the brink of *this* unsayable, experience-situated self, and an impending jaunt into *that* unsayable, *adjacent* experience-situated self. Going with, the core of healing, is mystical insofar as it can never be thought nor said, and only "be-d," only done; insofar as it is not achieved through having the right thoughts, but rather, that the right thoughts (and words) are had through achieving *it*; insofar as language is a failed medium to delineate what it is or how to achieve it. Going with is not a consequence but a version of materialization.

Implications: The Meaning of Therapeutic

The most important implication of "going with" is that it defines "a therapeutic encounter" not by any particular intervention, any particular language, any particular tone. In fact, it mandates entering into each encounter as if it has no necessary relationship with others. Any encounter might be related to a previous encounter, and any thought might be discussed in terms of previous thoughts, but only if this kind of dialogue comes to the fore. What's more, the criterion for "rightness"—i.e., the rightness of the therapist's thought and speech—is not strictly a matter of content. As "rightness" is a matter of *being with* the patient *where they are*, there is no utterance, no combination of words that is ruled out because it doesn't fit some conceptual criteria for "therapeutic." From this scheme, what's therapeutic is not predetermined; but if the reader understands me completely, what's therapeutic *is not determinable*. The dialogue that follows from sharing the other's coordinates in the intrinsic world is by definition therapeutic, whether it means receiving someone with complete empathy, needling them for a ridiculous idea, cracking an absurd joke, or offering a terribly hard-to-hear interpretation.

In these moments of togetherness in the intrinsic, nothing outside of the exchange holds any power to act as a criterion for *therapeutic*—not empirical knowns; not theories; not self-styled authorities of any kind; not norms; not sanctioned ways of delivering therapy; not something a scientist or teacher told you; not something your parents told you; definitely not something you read in a book (including this one); and not something of which you convinced yourself last month. These moments are the death of all things a-priori. Observations about life and therapy that have preceded these moments, and therefore might seem to "inform," possess *no power to inform*. Likewise, observing such moments after the fact, as a means of "confirming or disconfirming" their "relative" or "actual" therapeutic value, holds no such confirmatory potential. Moreover, neither the utility nor the authority of a therapeutic encounter is given by the clinician's level of expertise, their reservoir of available facts, or their fluency with elaborate case conceptualizations, all of which accrue as a matter of *time*. That is, we'd expect an 80-year-old clinician to have more of each than a 25-year-old, and we'd expect a psychoanalyst to have more of each after finishing five years at the institute—and we'd be right.

But meetings between patients and therapists do not garner their relative power, not fundamentally anyway, from anything related to time. They garner their power from something in the *right here*, something that is not made any easier or harder to find as a matter of what has come before it or what will come after it. An exchange propelled not by thinking about the other's subjectivity but rather by finding it holds authority unto itself, as it has dropped the construction of reality for reality, and the elaboration of experience for experience. Contact is the sole authority because it yields encounters moved not by *thinking about* the other's subjectivity but, somehow, by *sharing it*.

Thus, the language of psychotherapy might consist of anything, but if we are appropriately *going with* in good faith, the associated and extemporaneous dialogical exchange will always be for the good. This approach thus does not aim itself at preestablished outcomes. Rather, it aims itself at truth, thereby happily detaching itself from not only a-priori interventions but *interventions period*. This approach does not believe in the application of predetermined force, aimed at yielding predetermined kinds of change, because it doesn't believe that such approaches effect meaningful change. In fact, it sees all of modern psychotherapy's plans and schemes to impact its patients as misguided, not because they hold no utility—they hold some in terms of the outcomes we've designated—but because they misunderstand reality. *Going with* into experience, joining the other, is the right therapeutic tack because it "works." What's essential to understand, though, is that it "works" because it is true, because it reflects the *realest thing*. Regardless of our theoretical loyalties or our preferred therapeutic concepts, when any clinician is at their *most* useful, they are so because they are engaged in a task that *most* reflects ultimate reality:

> There is an ocean of experience, every drop of which we share, entirely. Although manifest interpersonal differences abound in every moment (i.e., how we think, feel, and act), we human beings are bonded by something that is the same, something that precedes every conceivable, observable, manifest, and non-manifest difference.

The best therapy is best not because it achieves "effectiveness," however we have constructed it. Rather, to the extent that it collapses two distinct experiences of this-ness—two previously separate consciousnesses into one—it achieves truth. The best therapy is itself the achievement of truth, and all therapy should be the pursuit of this truth because in finding it the most important things emerge. In *going with*, the therapist finds the experience of the patient within themselves, thereby eradicating all difference. When this happens, therapist and patient find themselves, together, in the same part of the ocean. This allows for a special kind of attunement, which yields the right thoughts and words, those marked not only by compassionate understanding, creativity, imagination, and productive spontaneity but also by increasing incorporation of logic and reason. "Knowledge transfer," so lampooned in Chapter 7, only works, it only lands, when there seems to be no discernable transfer—when self and other are at one. Similarly, real insight can happen when the real facts of the matter can be seen and put to use, but inconvenient or difficult facts are only necessarily acknowledged, admitted to, and accepted from this position.

Though it might sound radical to most of the field, which is taken with psychological science and its utilitarian-driven methods, all that is therapeutic grows from letting the patient take the lead. Even if in speech and dialogue we set in motion this or that exchange, which we certainly will, such initiations must follow from first having followed the patient into the intrinsic. This is not the prevailing way. By way of scientific knowing, many in our field assign themselves a very simple and manifest therapeutic mission: make depressed people less depressed, anxious people less anxious, and so on. And because they also claim knowledge of the exact route to these outcomes, what else would they do, except fearlessly lead the way? They say, with good intentions, "I know all about cognitive distortions and behavioral activation. Take my hand and come with me!" But this approach is marked by fear. Lending our expert hand to others and forging a path for them is not the healing agent. It is self-protective and even self-aggrandizing. We know much less than we are willing to admit about other human beings, even after an hour-long, diagnostic interview in which we fit them to our favorite constructs. If we were braver and more respectful, we would position our ignorance square in the middle of our work—it would *define* our work.

The most healing thing contained in this world is one person's readiness, *even eagerness*, to take the hand of the other, not in order to bring them somewhere specific, predetermined, and fashioned from one's own expertise; but instead, to go wherever they happen to be—willingly, without alarm, and of essential importance, without a single shred of pretense. Psychotherapy is accepting an invitation to a dance that has no predictable steps. It's a dance without a script, and it should be. For this reason, it is not a job for the fearful, for the proud, or for the righteous; it is not a job for the prescriptive or for the expert; but above all, it is not a job for the certain. The outstretched arm, which is essential to human healing, has a very specific meaning. It does not reach out in order to pull people into new ways of being, to educate them on who they are or what they need, or to inundate them, amid sanctimony, with one's own precious perspectives. The outstretched arm reaches out in order to be pulled in. It doesn't say "come with me." It says "I'll come with you. I'll dance with you in *whatever is*, in whatever *happens to now be*." On its face, psychotherapy looks like a therapist meeting the patient in the world of thought, language, and ideas—and as the reader will see in Volume II, it must be that, superficially. But there is much going on underneath the dialogue of the card game.

On the Failure of Methods

The mechanisms of action we cite in science—our rules for how things work—are rules for how the observable world works, by definition. For what they target, they are usually good rules, often accurate and clarifying. But these same rules cannot accurately explain or represent the experience of going with; as it is unintelligible to thought and the verbal elaboration that comprise "mechanisms," it is not governed by rules (where rules are stable propositions). What's more, *there is no* correlate that signifies that it has been fulfilled, except perhaps one: for patient and therapist, it often comes with a simple yet engrossing feeling of *realness.* In fact, every therapy session, even every moment of every therapy session, might be best thought of as containing some gradation of this quality; and not surprisingly, the sessions—and moments—in which this quality is most concentrated are most helpful. At bottom, the relative presence of this quality, but also the relative ease of its accretion might well be the whole game of psychotherapy.

And if it were the whole game, psychotherapy research would be permanently obstructed from finding the *thing* it is looking for (i.e., the mechanism) because the *thing* it is so hellbent on finding *wouldn't be a thing at all.* It would be an emergent, experiential property of dyadic interaction, somehow co-created by patient and therapist, forever confined to the air between them, which awakens the intrigue of the patient, propelling them, whether prudently or rabidly, into an exploration of all they might be. Were this the so-called "mechanism," psychotherapy research would be misguided to precisely the extent it assumes the mechanism at the heart of change is identifiable, conceptualizable, and delineable—to precisely the extent it assumes the mechanism at the heart of change could be made visible with concepts. The mechanism I am suggesting here could never be a "thing in itself" to be seamlessly observed, pursued, or taught.

What's more, while observation into therapeutic mechanisms has gotten us somewhere, it has also gotten us nowhere. For example, if what *really helped people* was contained in the specific utterances, behaviors, and responses—the specific interventions—we train each other to use, those necessarily derived from all that is visible, thinkable, formulable, therapy would look very different in one glaring way: our sanctioned interventions would "work" with near-perfect predictability. We would know whether they would effect change before implementing them. This is what it means for something to work and to know *how* something works. Each time I put gas in my car, for example, I can count on driving for several hours at leisure, with virtually no risk that the "filling up intervention" failed. But this doesn't apply in the domain of psychotherapy, does it?

The reason it doesn't is that the intervention itself, whatever its content, whatever our verbal explanations as to what inspired it, whatever came from it, is not what effects change. We all already know this. We know therapist utterances do not "work" because they contain X *word*, because they adhere to *theory* Y, because they are informed by Z *fact*, or even because they followed logically from that last thing the patient said. What we don't already know, because we are unwilling to (i.e., what we are too fearful and proud to know), is that entire conversations work, our contributions and those of our patients, because they are had at a certain *point in space* within the intrinsic world, one where division of all kinds—between self and other, this-ness and that-ness, current and ocean—simply dissolve into "no-otherness," which is an ineffable sense, altogether defiant of verbal capture.

Thus, our field's method for crafting interventions is flawed. All of our a-priori interventions earn *all of their shape* and earn *all of their validity* as a function of the very same process that, in therapy, distances us from patients: the representation of experience. They flow from that which can be mapped *about experience*. They are true, given the grounds on which they rest, but that ground is not only shaky; it's not even the same ground on which human harm *actually* exists: *actual* subjectivity. The *true* criterion for the "right intervention" is something less observable than our protocols would have us think. Whatever it is, it is made from *this* exchange with *this* person in *this* moment. Since there is no experiential corollary for *these kinds* of exchanges with *these kinds* of people in *these* kinds of moments, any criterion for "right intervention" that might come from such a method (e.g., where N=100), is a soothing mirage. It obviates the psychotherapist's truest, most hazardous task: to brazenly *go with* the other into that which grips them, whatever it is, which also exists, unavoidably and often more threateningly, in oneself.

The manifestation of "going with" is playing cards, simple talking, but it is talking in a different key; and as mysterious sounding as anything, it's talking from a different world—the truest, most intrinsic one. This version of talk permits us to say anything to people, including the most important things, the most human and personal things, things that do not generally find their way into protocols made for mobs of people. Now, the reader can appreciate my joyful dismissal of predetermined interventions. There is only one intervention, and its eventual form cannot be known ahead of time as it depends fully on the experience of self now gripping the other. The only intervention is to find the patient in the self, to find the other in the self, and to talk from a place of the deepest known reality: sameness. This is, always has been, and always will be the most powerful "intervention" known to mankind. What's more, when any of our concocted interventions have worked, they have worked because they were undergirded by this intervention—the truest, simplest, oldest, most powerful one.

What is a Therapist?

What can be said with certainty is that people are differentially adept at "going with" other people. What seems most associated with the ability to locate another's coordinates in the ocean is one's own practice with the ocean within. This needs to be said clearly if we want to be at all honest about psychotherapy. As stated in the first pages of this book, without an intimate understanding of the storm, a mission to find the other will only necessarily bring shipwreck. When one has committed to traversing all that exists within them, the more readily the other's whereabouts will materialize. Going with is a posture of loving openness, I think, achieved particularly by people who have journeyed within relentlessly, uncontrollably, and probably without much choice, thereby having found that internal experience is *nothing* if not shared, and psychical improvement is *nothing* if not experiential contact.

Because a clinician's main job is to expand the consciousness of the other via the embrace of more *experiences of self*, a clinician whose own consciousness is restricted is less likely to help. To the extent that a clinician cannot join the other in *what it's like*, only superficial gains can be made, regardless of the conceptual scheme (i.e., therapeutic modality) from which they are working. This, obviously, places an immeasurable burden on therapists with respect to their own relationship with themselves. It could be said that they must be well-acquainted with themselves, but this description is too refined, too soulless. What they must really know of themselves is that they are both saint and villain, both foolish and wise, both erudite and barbaric, both forgiving and vengeful. But more than that, those most prepared to go anywhere the patient happens to be have come to see the search for the ocean, the expedition into internal life, as an end in itself, regardless of whatever it turns up. It is not a utilitarian pursuit meant to improve existence; it is itself the improvement of existence.

Therapists most prepared to go anywhere with the other embody what is perhaps the strangest of human dualities. I feel very lucky to have been trained by many who have been cut from precisely this cloth (and I don't know that training in clinical psychology would have worked for me, had it been different). What's more, I now spend as much professional time as I can with this type. These are the people who are, at once, the least faint of heart and the most tenderhearted. This kind of person is completely awake. Somehow, they are *least blind* to anything that is real, even if what's real is painful, and *most open* to the inordinate difficulty of coming to reality. In blending an aggressive strength with a tender compassion, this kind of clinician grasps both the *absolute requirement* that we human beings illude ourselves about what we are (lest we suffer in ways we cannot bear) and the *absolute requirement* that we disillusion ourselves, eventually (lest we suffer permanently).

Revisiting This Book's First Question: What is a Changing Mind?

People can relinquish useless and harmful knowns and narratives (i.e., reality criteria), even those that are desperately clung to, like the side of a cliff standing between them and sure death would be (Chapter 3). Everything on the taken-for-granted path of our cognition—ranging from our manners of attending, perceiving, reasoning, and attributing, to the contents of conscious thought these processes produce—can be altered.

This is done by growing the experiences of self in which one is invested, by expanding the quality of this-ness that defines one's subjectivity; as this is the *very stuff* of one's unconceptualizable conceptualizing apparatus, growing it lends diversity to the conceptualizations it finds. In having available more experiences of self (i.e., more consciousness), cognitive processes—attention, perception, interpretation—become less indebted to any single one (or few), thereby becoming freer. In turn, cognition acquires more paths and ultimately more destinations—more conceptions of what the world *might be*. In turn, things that were always there but never attended to, perceived, or thought about come bounding into view. One sees with one's own mind altruism where there was once only instrumentalism (less cynicism); malice where there was once only ignorance (less naivete); fairness where there was once only corruption (more nuance). The whole complicated world, its paradoxes and contradictions, its wickedness and divinity, comes out of hiding. Yes, people can certainly know new things in their conscious minds, but the mind is not the vehicle; it's the red herring. *Knowing anew* is borne of being more of that which one really is—being more ocean and less current—which affords cognition the freedom it needs to see reality in the most accurate form *cognition* can possibly see it: as unrelenting, infinite, beautiful complexity.

With respect to the process of psychotherapy, it is often a good sign when people lack great explanations for the conscious changes they observe in themselves. In fact, it might be the primary sign of real and true change because changes in an unconceptualizable realm cannot be uttered—they can only happen. Thus, when noticed, they bring with them less reified sense-making. Patient descriptions of real change are often not-so-neatly packaged, a little bit dreamy, vague, even impressionistic and ungrounded. In the way they are conveyed, the listener has the distinct sense that something has happened for which there are no great words—and there aren't.

The Strange Superiority of Silence over Science

If any psychotherapy has the look of the one described at the outset of this chapter, defined by a lively and meaningful back and forth, something has already gone right. Regardless of 1) what appears to be taking place; 2) how that which is taking place would be conceptualized by either patient and therapist; or 3) the "treatment modality" within which it is allegedly taking place, effective psychotherapy is effective because it touches the investments the patient has made in the intrinsic world. Human healing is that which affords one the opportunity to investment in more experiences of self, to make contact with more of consciousness, and thereby, to become attentionally, perceptually, and cognitively freer. From there, minds change, knowns change, worlds change, and lives change.

The basic aim of psychotherapy—to change the mind of the other—involves contacting, intervening into, and expanding that which can never be known as a thing, that which can never take a defined form, that which can never be plainly viewable: the very this-ness populating the other's subjectivity, which follows from the investments he or she has made in the intrinsic world. This is a mark that will not be brought into the therapeutic crosshairs by conscious, devoted thought, but rather by a willingness to surrender to being gripped by something. Because psychotherapy's is one that neither therapist nor patient can conceive, in treatments that have gone right, both therapist and patient have hit a target that neither can see, one that somehow exists outside of all that is accessible to cognition. Were this proposition taken aboard, it could quiet psychotherapy debates in the most literal sense as it would reduce them to mere noise. Everyone describing therapeutic mechanisms is talking about a thing that no one can say (including me).

When we are talking about what changed a person, we are *representing changes* that took place in subjectivity *as represented*. But remember, the representation of subjectivity was no one's problem in the first place—subjectivity was. When thought cannot represent that which most makes a subject, how could it represent that which has changed one? The mechanism for changes to inexpressible first-person experience belongs forever to the inexpressible. This is to say that if something changed the intrinsic world of the other (i.e., the pattern of their intrinsic investments), then something changed *from within* a domain that will not be said. Thus, the psychotherapeutic mechanism by which one's investments actually grow is said most accurately with silence.

Loving *is* Going With *is* Knowing Rightly

Contemporary clinical psychology is decidedly disenchanted with processes that defy conceptualization, and thus sanctions methods of knowing about people that are much more concrete and formulaic than the one laid out in this volume. Nonetheless, I would like to propose that in the moment before a patient sits down across from us, we happily dispense with all such methods. Of crucial importance, however, mine is no recommendation for clinicians to give themselves free rein to say and do anything—quite the opposite, actually.

The core of the method I am offering is singularly and inescapably moral. No matter what we happen to be saying, thinking, or doing in a given therapy session, there is a deeper task on which our sights must always be set. This is perhaps the only thing from which we therapists should never, ever stray. It's the first and last rule of psychotherapy. It goes like this: we must always be committed to improving the quality of relationship that the other has with themselves. In practice, this means going with the other and thereby helping them to expand their investments, so that more of themselves becomes available to them, not to be dealt with, eradicated, or altered but to be touched and further cultivated. This is the intention of all intentions; it constitutes an ethical galaxy unto itself; and it is the very definition of human love.

INDEX

human healing xv, xvii, 166, 183–184, 201, 205

intractable self 156–158; and moral change 164–165
intrinsic world of being; as relational binding agent 20–22; defiance of cognitive representation 186; depiction of *168*; introduction to 16–17; of 22–23; *see also* ocean of experience
investing process; detailed explanation of 106–111, 169–170; introduction to 25–27

Kierkegaard, S. 23
knowing; and empiricism 53–55; and evidence 51–53; anew 65, 115, 204–205; as a pursuit of safety 85–89; the experience of 49–50; the misattribution of 64–65; -derivatively, 136; what we already know 90–96
Kohut, H. 23

language; overvaluing of 37–42, 122, 179–181
loss and loathing; as obstructions to change 145
love; and morality 105–106, 142–144; as deepest quality of subjectivity 26–27, 105; as; essential to psychotherapy 28, 116, 165, 184, 206; role in investing process 26–27, 106–108

material world 5; shape of 151; losses in 161
motivation 73–74; failure of paradigms of impact to account for 69, 72
Mysticism; as an encounter xxiv–xxix; as an idea 23–24; in therapeutic action 197–198

no otherness 202

ocean of experience 99–102; 108; 135; 159; 169–170, 192; as ultimate reality 200; defiance of cognitive representation 186; depiction of *168*; relationship with moral progress 164; relationship with psychic progress 183; *see also* intrinsic world of being

omniscience; in society 15; in psychotherapy 168

perception; felt accuracy of 94–96; perceiver in 92–94

reality criteria 94–98, 171–172; depiction of *168*; development of 104–112; reinforcement of 174; relationship with experiential currents 99–100; relationship with experiences of self 111–116; therapeutic effects on 114–116
representation; of that which can only be done 58–61; of that which can only be experienced 16–17, 21, 187
restoration *see* human healing
right knowing 42, 146–147, 206
Rogers, C. 23

Schopenhauer, A. 23
self-reflection; necessity of 2–10
silence 63, 93, 205–206
soul 28, 121; an independent 8–9; and going with 195; gift to 7; the other's 88; assessment by 107–108; psychology's loss of 121; pursuit of and by 161
striving mind *see* cognitive striving

tenderness 110
therapist 1, 203–204; person of xvii; soulfulness of 132; 204
this-ness; as an experiential quality 65, 109–113, 169–171; as the door to the other 189, 192; impossible complexity of 190–192; role in change 177–184, 186–187, 193, 194, 197, 200, 202, 204, 205; role in cognitive processes 113–116, 170–172, 178–181 ; *see also* experience of self; *see also* unconceptualizable conceptualizing apparatus

unconceptualizable conceptualizing apparatus 58–61, 103–104, 113; idiosyncrasy of 62–63; in misattribution of knowing 64–65; *see also* experience of self; *see also* this-ness
understanding 58–63; versus having an understanding 75–77